# PLANT-BASED DIET FOR BEGINNERS

*LEARN HOW TO KEEP YOUR BODY ENERGIZED ALL DAY WITH HEALTHY READY TO GO MEALS USING THE NEWEST 4 WEEKS PLANT-BASED DIET MEAL PLAN AND HOW TO STOP EMOTIONAL EATING*

# Table of Contents

# Introduction

Whether you are already convinced that plant-based eating is the best way to go, or just plain curious about this increasingly popular diet, this book will guide you in understanding the what's, how's and why's of a plant-based diet.

Plant-based eating is not too restrictive nor is it difficult to follow. You will find an array of easy, affordable and inspirational ideas on how to include more plant-based foods into your diet—from main hearty meals and quick creative lunches to refreshing juices and smoothies and fun tasty desserts.

In contrast, most fad diets are very motivating at first but eventually fail because eliminating and restricting food groups may end up backfiring by increasing your risks of getting sick.

Still not sure if you can commit to eating plant-based foods100 percent? No need to worry. The following chapters will show you in detail how you do not need to approach a plant-based diet with an all-or-nothing attitude. Rest assured that every step you take is a step closer to lowered risks of developing chronic diseases, and higher energy levels through a plant-based diet that you can stick with for the rest of your longer and healthier life.

The availability of the variety of diet plans has made the choice of a perfect diet plan very perplexing. Almost all dietitians and nutritionists across the world recommend diet plans that support fresh and whole foods and restrict processed foods. The Plant-Based Diet is based on these unanimously preferred foods.

Plant-based diet patterns focus on foods predominantly from plants, including fruits, vegetables, nuts, oils, seeds, whole grains, beans, and legumes. This diet does not make you strictly a vegetarian or vegan who is not allowed to eat meat or dairy. Instead, you have to consume more of your foods from plant sources. This introduction emphasizes the importance and benefits of a plant-based diet. It will clear away all of your doubts and reservations regarding the plant-based diet plan.

You may still be reluctant about following the plant-based diet if you are not familiar with its benefits. This section will give you an idea about the various ways in which the plant-based diet will help your body and allow you to improve your overall state of health.

This is a primary benefit that draws many people toward this diet. Obesity and other weight issues have been increasing in alarming proportions over the years. This can be countered by making the right dietary choices and changing your lifestyle for the better. The plant-based diet helps you do that. The diet will help you consume a lot of fiber -and reduce the amount of processed foods you consume. This is automatically a way to shed extra weight from your body. Studies show that people following the plant-based diet lose more weight compared to those who follow a more animal food-based diet.

Other than the personal benefits you reap, you also have to appreciate the fact that this diet is good for the planet. The modern-day diet rich in processed foods and animal-based foods have a very negative effect on the environment over the last decade. A plant-based diet will allow you to leave a much smaller environmental footprint. Sustainability is allowed when you follow the plant-based diet. This will help in the reduction of greenhouse gas emissions, land use as well as water wastage. All of these factors play a big role in global warming.

As you can see, the plant-based diet has numerous benefits that will help you lose excess weight, reduce the risk of various diseases, and also help you lead a much more environmentally conscious life. All of this should definitely motivate you to try out the wholesome plant-based diet.

# Chapter 1: Macros and Micros of

# plant based plan

A plant-based diet plan is a complete change of lifestyle, which is why it does not follow any strict rules for its configuration. You simply have to cut off animal-based foods entirely from your diet. Listed below are a few factors for a plant-based diet plan:

1. Eliminate animal-based foods.

2. Consume plants like seeds, legumes, fruits, veggies, nuts, and whole grains abundantly.

3. Emphasize more on the whole, natural, or minimally processed foods.

4. Eat locally-sourced and organic food when possible.

5. Cut off refined foods, including white flour, processed oils, and added sugars.

Most of the above traits are also found in vegetarian and vegan diet plans, which is why the whole-food plant-based diet is easily confused with them. But, trust us, they are different. A vegan diet eliminates all animal-related foods, including seafood, dairy, honey, meat, and poultry. On the other hand, vegetarian diets exclude meat and poultry but typically allow seafood, dairy products, eggs, and honey.

Contrary to them, the whole-food plant-based diet plan is more flexible and forgiving. The food is mostly plant-based, but you can also eat animal-based products in moderation. The extent of animal-related foods in your diet plan depends on your personal choice of entirely not eating them or consuming them in small amounts. In short, a whole-food plant-based diet plan is comprised of plant-based foods with a minimal amount of animal-related products and processed foods.

Plant foods possess most of the primary nutrients and their substituents, which are as follows: Protein Proteins are composed of amino acids, which are an essential source of energy in the human body. Quinoa contains all essential amino acids and is a rich source of proteins. Plants, such as nuts, beans, lentils, and soy seeds are a great source of proteins.

## Vitamin B12

Vitamin B12 is abundantly acquired via fish, meat, dairy products, and eggs. However, a plant-based diet makes sure to make vitamin B12 available through fortified yeast, cereals, and soy milk. The deficiency of vitamin B12 causes anemia and nerve damage, so the followers of this diet can take supplements to avoid its lack.

### Iron

The iron is an essential mineral that carries blood oxygen to different parts of the body. The plant food, which is an excellent source of iron, are dark green vegetables (spinach, kale, peas), whole grains, bread, nuts, seeds, dried beans, and cereals. The iron obtains from plant sources absorbs less as compared to the animal source. The absorption of plant-based iron can be increased with vitamin C.

## Vitamin C

Vitamin C is vital for humans and oranges, kiwis, broccoli, strawberries, and tomatoes are good plant sources of vitamin C.

## Vitamin D

Vitamin D is required for a healthy immune system, bones, and muscles. Plant sources of vitamin D are almond milk and some cereals.

### Omega-3- Fatty acid

Omega 3 fatty acids play an essential role in reducing the risk of heart diseases and improving the immune system. Fatty fish and other seafood are the best sources for this nutrient. Omega 3 fatty acids can be obtained through various plant sources, including chia seeds, organic canola oil, flaxseeds, and flaxseed oil.

### Zinc

Zinc is known to strengthen the immune system, assist wound healing, and maintaining blood sugar levels. Plant sources of zinc include tofu, whole grains, peas, tempeh, nuts, and lentils. Phyllates is a compound in plants that inhibits the absorption of zinc, so it is best to soak plants overnight.

### Calcium

Bones and teeth are composed mainly of calcium. Calcium also improves nerves, muscles, and heart. Soy milk, almond, tofu, kale, bok choy, and broccoli are the best sources of calcium.

The first important tip is to get rid of meaty thoughts and personalize your plant-based diet plan by customizing your favorite recipes into this diet. You must try some new recipes with a different style for breakfast, lunch, dinner, snacks, and beverages. Your aim should be to stay as healthy as you could by abstaining from meat and dairy.

# Chapter 2: The Benefits

One of the main reasons that urge people to switch to a plant-based diet is the fact that it has so many wonderful and amazing health benefits. When you cut out all of the bad, processed food from your diet and replace it instead with whole, unrefined, and carefully-sourced plant products, you feel the benefits almost immediately. In fact, the healthy change is really what keeps most people on the diet. There is so much motivation to stay within the parameters of a plant-based diet when you are actually feeling better, healthier, and have more energy and stamina. Who would want to go back to eating unhealthily and feeling slow and sluggish after getting a taste of what your life on plant-based foods is like? And as an added bonus, you can set your conscience at ease and know that you are taking the steps towards making a better, more protected planet. The plant-based diet is without a doubt one of the most environmental ways of eating you could choose.

There is no denying that we are in the midst of a crisis of chronic diseases like high cholesterol, diabetes, and high-blood pressure. Many people blame the almost universal shift to eating foods that are processed and animal-sourced like refined grains, sugar, salt, meat, oil, dairy, soda, and eggs. Most of the time, these foods are high in fat and low in nutritional value but we keep reaching for them all the same. However, there most certainly is hope.

Plant-based diets are becoming much more mainstream and popular amongst people looking to improve their health and lengthen their lifespans. There are so much more products on the market geared towards helping people achieve a healthy, plant-based diet lifestyle than there used to be. Nowadays, you can easily find entire restaurants devoted to serving healthy plant-based meals and health food stores are a dime a dozen. It is easier than ever to switch to a plant-based diet. And that most certainly is good news for you.

We know for a fact that a plant-based diet is a healthier choice than eating lots of processed foods and animal products. Extensive research has been done on this topic. In one study, researchers used vegetarians who had lapsed from their diets as their main focus group. They found that people who used to subscribe to a vegetarian diet but fell out of it and began to eat meat at least once a week experienced an extremely raised risk of heart disease, stroke, diabetes, and weight gain. Studying them for 12 years after they transitioned away from a vegetarian diet, researchers found that life-expectancy was decreased as well. In studies where researchers put certain groups afflicted with diseases like heart disease, high cholesterol, or high blood pressure on an interventional plant-based diet, they found significant increases in satisfaction and health. These groups placed on plant-based diets reported that they were happier with their diet, had increased energy, better digestion, improved sleep, and overall better general and mental health. A plant-based diet has been proven to lower body weight, reduce sugar levels, and aids the body in controlling cholesterol levels. It also helps deal with your emotional and mental health. Many people who switch to a plant based diet claim to experience a lessening of afflictions such as anxiety, fatigue, and depression. It gives many a greater sense of well-being and makes day-to-day functioning easier and more enjoyable.

Therefore, a plant-based diet is a kind of foolproof way to lower your cholesterol. High cholesterol and blood pressure are dangerous factors that lead to heart disease, the number one killer of adults in the United States. A plant-based diet thus lowers your risk of heart disease because it ensures that you are putting better, healthier foods into your body that will not make your blood pressure and cholesterol levels sky rocket like some of the other fatty, processed foods and animal products out there.

Followers of a plant-based diet also experience better blood sugar levels. The simplest way to combat high blood sugar is to consume more fiber as is slows the absorption of sugar into the bloodstream. Plant foods and whole grains are incredibly high in fiber while animal products have been proven to raise blood sugar to unhealthy and at times dangerous levels. More balanced blood sugar helps prevent against type 2 diabetes and results in a much healthier life. Whole foods that are nutritious and low in fat also greatly decrease your risk of cancer. Some animal products such as cured meats are thought to be linked to the development of certain cancers. With a plant-based diet, your chances of having cancer are much lowered than someone who does not subscribe to a plant-based diet. It is for these many reasons that many doctors actually champion the plant-based diet and recommend it to patients who are overweight or afflicted with high cholesterol, high blood pressure, or other cardiovascular troubles. Plant-based diets have been shown time and time again to be economical and low-risk ways to make a significant change in one's health for the better. Switching to a plant-based diet may help lower the body mass index (BMI) in addition to blood pressure and cholesterol levels. Because of this, patients may need to take less medications in order to treat their illnesses, thus cutting out unnecessary expenses and the need to take many pills. All of these heart healthy benefits also manifest themselves in the form of weight management and appetite control, all of which we will delve further into in the next chapter.

When you begin to feel immensely healthier due to all the benefits of a plant-based diet, it is inevitable that your mental and emotional health will follow along. Many people notice improved sleeping patterns after making the switch. Not only do they sleep more regularly, the sleep deeper and better. Sleep is so important to our mental and physical health and unfortunately, it is usually one of the first things we sacrifice in our daily lives. There are deadlines to be met, tasks to be completed, and things to do-it can all get overwhelming. When do we have time to sleep? And when we do, is it a good sleep? Switching to a plant-based diet can really help you get in control of your sleep and maximize the actual benefits of your pillow time. Eating plant-based makes the body a well-oiled machine and as such, it becomes more able to recharge itself efficiently. Therefore, you get the most out of your precious, valuable time for sleep. Better sleep can lead to a significant increase in the quality of one's mental health. A good night's sleep elevates mood and boosts energy so that you can be more productive and motivated during the day.

In addition to the many medical benefits of switching to a plant-based diet, there are also some truly powerful and indisputable cosmetic benefits as well. Many studies have shown that there is a significant and strong link between the consumption of dairy products like milk, butter, or cheese, and undesirable skin conditions like acne, eczema, and early signs of aging. Milk contains many similar properties to the hormone testosterone due to other hormones like progesterone making their way into the milk. It is thought that these hormones stimulate the oil glands of the skin, especially the face. An excess of sebum, or oil, is produced and thus acne occurs. This excess oil clogs your pores and can lead to other troublesome skin blemishes such as blackheads and whiteheads. This continuous cycle of clogged pores, blemishes, and acne takes a lot out of your skin and can cause scarring and stress. This can lead to signs of premature aging and skin loses its elasticity and vitality. Many people who switch to a plant-based diet notice an incredibly rapid improvement in the condition of their skin. People who have suffered from acne and started eating plant-based foods have noticed their skin clear significantly. This is in no way by chance. Cutting out or greatly reducing dairy can really help give your skin a new lease on life. If you are struggling with acne and have tried nearly everything under the sun such as harsh chemicals, expensive facials and skin treatments, or countless different brands claiming to heal your skin problems, something as simple as a plant-based diet may be the answer you've been searching for.

Followers of a plant-based diet have also raved about the excellent anti-aging benefits of the diet. Collagen, something our bodies naturally produce in abundance when we are young, is the key factor of what makes skin supple, resilient, firm, and have elasticity. As we get older, collagen production slows and our skin suffers as a result, becoming prone to sagginess and thinness. While this is a natural and inevitable part of life, collagen loss does not have to be so drastic as we age. A plant-based diet has been proven to boost collagen in your body by providing all of the important nutrients and amino acids that make up collagen and how it is produced. In a sense, subscribing to a plant-based diet is kind of like taking a dip in the fountain of youth! Fruits and vegetables like kale, broccoli, asparagus, spinach, grapefruit, lemons, and oranges are chock-full of vitamin C which is an extremely important component in producing the amino acids that make up collagen. The kind of lean protein found in nuts is important in keeping collagen around, adding to skin cell longevity and resilience. Red vegetables like tomatoes, beets, and red peppers all contain lycopene which is a kind of antioxidant that protects skin from the sun while simultaneously increases collagen production. Foods rich in zinc such as certain seeds and whole grains also promote collagen because the mineral repairs damaged cells and reduces inflammation. So many of the plant-based staples contain incredible amounts of all these collagen-boosting nutrients that you do not even have to go out of your way to seek them out. It is all right there in front of you! Looking and feeling younger has never been so easy. It really does start with the internal to make the external radiant and glowing, outer beauty starts from within.

In short, there are no two ways about it - switching to a plant based diet is good for your heart, your health, your mind, and even your physical appearance! The facts of the matter are undeniable. Plant foods contain so many of the incredibly good nutrients that our bodies need to function properly. Making these foods a priority and centering your meals around them rather than just eating vegetables as an occasional side dish or a piece of fruit every now and then makes a huge difference in your health. By eating a diet heavy on meat, dairy, and other animal products and processed foods, it is easy to miss out on the wonderfully beneficial vitamins, minerals, antioxidants, and other nutrients that are in fruits, vegetables, legumes, tubers, grains, nuts, and seeds. Switching to a plant-based diet gives you the opportunity to obtain all of these healthful ingredients that will without a doubt lead you to a better, more fulfilling life.

A plant-based diet has significant benefits of improving health and being eco-friendlier. Some of the benefits are as follows:

Weight Loss and Overall Improved Health Obesity is one of the significant health issues faced by the majority of people these days, ranging from children to old. Proper diet changes can lead to radical weight loss, which would be promising and long-lasting. Various studies report that effective weight loss can be achieved with the help of plant-based diet plans.

The plant-based diet plan is ideal for weight loss, as it is rich in proteins and fiber, limits processed foods, and forbids refined grains, soda, candy, fast food, and added sugars. According to a few research reports, plant-based diet followers lose weight more quickly as compared to non-plant-based diet followers. Weight loss from a plant-based diet plan is quite long-lasting with improved health.

Beneficial in Various Health Issues In addition to weight loss, a plant-based diet helps to reduce the menaces of numerous chronic health conditions.

Cardiac Conditions The foremost benefit of a plant-based diet plan is that it keeps the cardiac health sound, depending upon the quality and types of the food in your diet plan. Research studies report that the risk of cardiac diseases was lower in those people who follow a plant-based diet that was rich in veggies, whole grains, nuts, fruits, and legumes, as compared to followers of other diets. Plant-based diet plans, including refined grains, sugary drinks, and fruit juices, are very unhealthy and contribute to severe cardiac complications. So, it is essential to follow a healthy plant-based diet plan.

Cancer Research studies report that a plant-based diet plan can avoid various forms of cancer. The risks of gastrointestinal and colorectal cancers are reported to be significantly reduced amongst plant-based diet followers.

Cognitive Decline According to some studies, Alzheimer's disease and cognitive decline can be prevented in adults with the help of diet plans high in veggie and fruit content due to a large number of antioxidants and other compounds. Consumption of more fruits and vegetables leads to a 20 percent lower risk of having dementia or cognitive impairment.

Diabetes In order to reduce the risk of contracting diabetes, one should consider following a plant-based diet plan. Followers of the plant-based diet plan mitigate the risk of having diabetes by 34 percent when compared to followers of other diets. Fifty percent reduction of type 2 diabetes was observed amongst the followers of Lacto-Ovo vegetarian and vegan diet plans. Blood sugar level control is highly improved in the diabetic followers of plant-based diet plans.

Eco-friendlier Diet In addition to benefits in health, a plant-based diet plan has proved to be advantageous for the ecosystem, as they have little effect on the environment as compared to other diet plan followers. A plant-based diet helps in the minimization of global warming, as it results in a 50-70 percent reduction in greenhouse gas emissions, land usage, and lower water usage. A plant-based diet also helps in boosting the economy due to lower dependency on unsustainable practices like factory farming and reduction in animal-based food.

# Chapter 3: The basics

## What Is Plant Based Diet?

A plant-based diet is not synonymous to a vegetarian or vegan diet. Although these terms are often used interchangeably, they are not the same.

A plant-based diet is focused on proportionately eating more foods primarily from plants and cutting back on animal-derived foods. However, it does not necessarily involve eliminating entire food groups and lean sources of protein. This means, those on a plant-based diet may still opt to eat some meat.

Going vegan, on the other hand, means being strictly against animal products in any form—from never eating meat and dairy products to not patronizing products tested on animals and not wearing animal products such as leather.

A healthy plant-based diet generally emphasizes meeting your nutritional needs by eating more whole plant foods, while reducing the intake of animal products. Whole foods refer to natural, unrefined or minimally refined foods. Plant foods consist of those that do not have animal ingredients such as meat, eggs, honey, milk and other dairy products.

In contrast, those on a vegetarian diet may still eat processed and refined foods. Vegetarians can even eat fast foods, junk food and other salty snacks guilt-free.

Once you get started with this diet, you will notice a huge difference in how you feel each day. From the time that you wake up in the morning, you will feel that you have more energy, and that you do not get tired as easily as before. You will also have more mental focus and fewer mood-related problems.

As for digestion, a plant-based diet is also said to improve how the digestive system works. In fact, dieters confirm fewer incidences of stomach pains, bloating, indigestion and hyperacidity.

Then there's the weight loss benefit that we cannot forget about. Since a plant-based diet means eating fruits, vegetables, and whole grains that have fewer calories and are lower in fat, you will enjoy weight loss benefits that some other fad diets are not able to provide.

Aside from helping you lose weight; it maintains ideal weight longer because this diet is easier to sustain and does not require elimination of certain food groups.

Don't worry about not getting enough nutrients from your food intake. This diet provides all the necessary nutrients including proteins, vitamins, minerals, carbohydrates, fats, and antioxidants. And again, that's because it does not eliminate any food group but only encourages you to focus more on plant-based food products.

## What to Eat and What to Avoid?

Foods Allowed on a Plant-Based Diet Plan Most of the people prefer to eat animal-based products for every meal. The focus of the plant-based diet plan is to make plant-based foods the primary food source. Consume animal-based foods in smaller quantities if you have a craving for them. Instead of making the animal-based foods the central part of the dish, use these foods, like seafood, meat, eggs, poultry, and dairy as a side dish. Below is a list of plant-based foods to make your choices easier.

Fruits: bananas, pears, berries, citrus fruits, pineapples, peaches, etc.

Veggies: peppers, broccoli, spinach, asparagus, tomatoes, kale, carrots, cauliflower, etc.

Whole grains: rolled oats, farro, barley, quinoa, brown rice pasta, brown rice, etc.

Starchy veggies: potatoes, butternut squash, sweet potatoes, etc.

Legumes: peas, peanuts, black beans, chickpeas, lentils, etc.

Plant-based milks (unsweetened): almond milk, cashew milk, coconut milk, etc.

Condiments: mustard, lemon juice, soy sauce, salsa, nutritional yeast, vinegar, etc.

Nuts, nut butters, and seeds: pumpkin seeds, sunflower seeds, tahini, cashews, almonds, macadamia nuts, natural peanut butter (sugar-free), etc.

Pork & beef: if possible, select pasture-raised or grass-fed.

Dairy products: if possible, choose organic dairy products from pasture-raised animals.

Seafood: if possible, pick wild-caught from sustainable fisheries.

### Foods to Avoid or Limit on the Plant-Based Diet Plan

The primary focus of a plant-based diet plan is to avoid as much artificially-produced food as possible and add natural food to your plate. Heavily processed foods are strictly prohibited in a plant-based diet plan. So, you must choose fresh foods while you are purchasing grocery items. Select the packaged food with the least amount of ingredients, in case you need to buy them necessarily. Below are listed the foods that need to be avoided on a plant-based diet plan: Added sugars and sweets: candy, soda, sugary cereals, pastries, sweet tea, table sugar, juice, cookies, etc.

Below are listed the foods that have to be restricted for a plant-based diet plan even if you include healthy animal-based products in your diet: Game meats Pork Sheep Beef Dairy Seafood Eggs Poultry

# Chapter 4: Planning the pantry

Unlike with other diet programs, with the plant-based diet, you don't have to worry too much about getting stared.

As you will find out for yourself, getting started is not that difficult because most likely, you are already eating most of what is required. There's a big chance that you will only need to make minimal changes in your diet.

Here are the steps on how to get started: Step # 1 – Write down your current diet Do not make any changes with your diet first. For the first week, record all the dishes and snacks that you eat throughout the day. This will show you what areas in your food habits are necessary to be changed, and which ones can be retained.

Step # 2 – Write down a menu based on this diet Once you're done with recording the past week's diet, you can now create your diet for the second week. Take note that you don't have to completely overhaul your diet immediately as this will make the transition too drastic and might not provide positive results.

Start avoiding some of the foods and drinks that are not encouraged in a plant-based diet. You should also start adding more fruits and vegetables to dishes that you love. For example, if you are fond of eating oatmeal in the morning, it would be a great idea to start packing it with bananas, apples and mangoes.

If you love snacking on yogurt, make it a point to stir in some blueberries or strawberries.

Step # 3 – Cut down on meat consumption Do not completely avoid all types of meat. But you just have to reduce intake slowly but surely. For instance, instead of eating steak with mashed potatoes on the side for dinner, why don't you try sautéing green beans with a few strips of beef and serve it with mashed potatoes on the side. This way, there are more vegetables than meat in your dish.

Step # 4 – Fill your pantry with healthy items It's a lot harder to adopt a healthy diet if you kitchen is filled with all sorts of junk foods. Discard the candies, sweet treats, sugary beverages and bags of chips that are in your pantry. Replace these with natural and healthy snacks like kale chips, whole grain bread slices, and fruit desserts.

What to Eat

Here's a list of all the foods and drinks that you should focus on while on a plant-based diet:

Fruits – Apples, bananas, blueberries, blackberries, pears, oranges, mangoes, avocados, pineapple, strawberries, raspberries

Vegetables – Spinach, tomatoes, carrots, cucumber, zucchini, potatoes, squash, broccoli, cauliflower, kale, cabbage

Whole grains – Brown rice, quinoa, oats, barley, whole wheat bread, whole wheat pasta

Legumes – Peanuts, beans, peas, chickpeas, lentils

Plant-based protein – Tempeh, tofu

Nuts – Almonds, walnuts, pistachios

Nut butters

Seeds – Sunflower seeds, flax seeds

Healthy oils – Olive oil, avocado oil, grapeseed oil

Herbs and spices

Water

Coffee

Tea

Smoothies

Fresh fruit or veggie juices

Now, here's a list of all the foods and drinks that you can consume but try to limit intake as much as possible.

Meat – Beef, pork, lamb

Poultry – Chicken, turkey

Seafood – Fish, shells, crabs, shrimp

Dairy products – Milk, cheese, yogurt

Processed meats - Bacon, sausage

What to Avoid

This one is a list of the foods and drinks that you would want to avoid as much as possible.

Fast food

Sweetened beverages

Refined grains – White bread, white rice, refined pasta

Packaged foods – Cookies, chips, cereals

TIPS

Make the transition for you easier using the following tips and strategies:

Make a meal planner

Write down a menu for the week or for the month so you don't have to worry about steering away from your healthy diet. It would be a good idea to make use of an online meal planner that you can access even when you're outside your home. But if you prefer to do it the traditional way, and write it on paper, that is a good idea too.

Eat small healthy snacks during the day

Doing this will keep you full longer and will reduce the possibility of getting tempted to eat foods that are not encouraged in a plant-based diet. If you are full, there's less tendency for you to crave for a huge slab of steak for instance.

Don't be too hard on yourself

Making a transition from one diet to another is always difficult and challenging. Do not expect yourself to be immediately comfortable with your new diet. It may take you longer than a week. It would probably require you at least a month to ease in to your new diet, even if this is not as restrictive as other types of diet.

Use meat as garnish

Instead of making it the centerpiece of your dish, use it as an "add-on". Instead of serving steak with a small amount of steamed veggies on the side, it would be better to turn things around and serve more steamed veggies and just a little amount of meat.

Use good fats

Make it a point to use only healthy fats like olive oil, avocados, nut butter and so on.

Have lots of salads

Salads are a great way to turn your regular diet into one that's plant-based. Not only that, these are extremely convenient to prepare and will only take you a few minutes to prepare. You won't have to spend a long time in the kitchen to cook an elaborate meal.

Satisfy cravings for sweets with fruits

There will always be those times when you will crave for something sweet. For some people, this usually happens after a meal. Do not deprive yourself. Instead, satisfy your craving the healthy way—eat fruits for dessert.

Follow these tips to ensure to have a smooth transition from your old diet into this new one. It may not be as challenging as with other diet programs, but of course, there will also be certain drawbacks that you would want to be prepared for.

Basic Shopping List

Shopping for a plant-based diet plan sounds tough, but it is pretty much easier. We are providing you with a list of foods that you can opt for while following the diet plan. You don't need to stick solely to this list; rather we recommend making changes to make the diet plan more versatile. The only thing to keep in mind is that it should be having plant-based ingredients. One more important thing to understand is that the formulation of products might change, so you have to keep a close eye on the labels on foods. The list includes the following: 1. Fresh Produce (Veggies and Fruits) You can have a wide variety of fresh vegetables and fruits. Go for various dark leafy green veggies. We recommend avoiding avocados if you have cardiac complications and eat more if you are aiming to lose weight.

2. Legumes and Beans You can enjoy all variants of lentils and dried beans. In case you opt for canned beans, prefer going for

no salt or low-sodium. If you are unable to find any no-salt-added beans, rinse the beans thoroughly before using them.

3. Seeds, Nuts, and Dried Fruits Don't go for nuts if you have cardiac complications and eat more of them if you wish to lose weight. In case you opt for nuts, every variant is better but prefer going for no-oil added or raw. Don't eat them by the handful as their fat content is high, and so is their calorie content, and it can make you overeat it. You can also use nut butter.

You can go for omega-3 rich flax and chia seeds for topping cereals and even replacing eggs in your baking recipes. The content should be 1 tbsp. of chia or ground flaxseed in addition to 3 tbsp of water, which is the equivalent of 1 egg. Whole flax seeds are hard to digest, so prefer going for ground flaxseed, or you can grind them in a coffee grinder before usage. Eat more seeds like pumpkin seeds, sesame, and sunflower seeds, etc.

Go for dried fruits, but keep in mind that they are not having any added sugar. One more important thing to remember is that that are having higher calories than fresh fruits. If you have a diabetic condition or are aiming to lose weight, prefer going for fresh fruits instead of dried ones. Moreover, avoid having dried banana chips as they are fried most of the time.

4. Frozen Fruits You can have all types of frozen veggies and fruits without having dairy ingredients or added oil.

You can also have a wide variety of whole-grain rice like long, medium, and short-grain, black, red, purple, wild, jasmine, and much more. You can have any type of rice, but not white rice on the plant-based diet plan.

You can have a wide array of whole-grain flours in your diet plan too. These include: • Whole wheat pastry flour • White whole wheat flour • Whole wheat flour • Oat Flour • Barley Flour • Amaranth Flour • Rye Flour • Spelt Flour • Kamut Flour Apart from these, you can also go for gluten-free flours if you are having any allergies to wheat. But it is important to read the labels carefully as various gluten-free flours are processed.

Mustards: You are not allowed to have high sugar honey mustard sauces.

Capers: You should rinse it before usage for minimizing the sodium content.

Olives: Go for olives that are not packed in oil, sparingly use them as they are very high in sodium.

Cheese Substitutes You should go for nutritional yeast for sprinkling purposes on pasta and even use it in recipes for adding a "cheesy" flavor to them. Special occasion's option includes: • Miyoko's Creamery cheeses (choose the no added oil varieties) • Miyoko's Creamery cheeses (choose the no added oil varieties) They are very high in fat, so you have to use them in a moderate manner.

# Chapter 5: Plant based foods that boost immunity and Plant based beauty treatments

## Plant based foods that boost immunity

This list includes plant and plant-based products such as:

- Fruits and vegetables

- Whole grains, cereals, and pseudo-cereals such as spelt, quinoa, and teff—all of which are high-protein options that are also great sources of complex carbs, B vitamins, and several minerals such as zinc, iron, potassium, to name a few, and fiber.

- Fermented and sprouted plant foods. This includes pickles, kimchi, Ezekiel bread, miso, natto, and tempeh.

- Nutritional yeast. This is a great protein supplement you can include in dishes as a substitute for cheese given its cheesy flavor.

- Seeds such as chia seeds, flax seeds, and hemp seeds which are good sources of protein and omega-3 fatty acids.

- Nuts and nut butters are great sources of fiber, magnesium, zinc, selenium, vitamin E, and iron. The unroasted and unblanched varieties are best.

- Legumes such as lentils, beans, and peas are great protein sources and increase nutrient absorption.

- Plant-based protein replacements. This includes tofu, tempeh, and seitan. They make great replacements for meat, fish, poultry, and eggs in recipes.

- Calcium-fortified plant milks and yogurts. These are a great replacement for milk and yogurt and help provide the recommended daily supplement of calcium. Try to get versions that have been fortified with vitamin B12 and D when possible.

## Plant based foods for beauty treatment

You are free to consume as many vegetables as you want. Most of the vegetables are low in calories and rich in dietary fiber, phytonutrients, antioxidants, minerals, and vitamins that your body needs. You can use fresh as well as frozen vegetables.

The vegetables you can include are avocados, artichokes, asparagus, bell peppers, beetroot, broccoli, cabbage, brussels sprouts, cauliflower, carrots, cherry tomatoes, celery, collard greens, eggplant, cucumber, corn, peas, green beans, olives, jalapenos, mushrooms, okra, radishes, pumpkins, potatoes, shallots, squash, fennel, onions, chilies, peppers, potatoes, sweet potatoes, rhubarb, sprouts, zucchini, turnips, yams, and parsnips. The greens you can include are kale, spinach, Swiss chard, bok choy, arugula, lettuce, mixed salad leaves, watercress, endives, and so on.

You can pretty much include any vegetables that you want, including any which haven't been mentioned in this list.

Fruits are rich in antioxidants, minerals, enzymes, vitamins, and other phytonutrients. They pretty much include all the good stuff that your body needs. The simple sugars present in fruits also give your body a quick boost of energy. You can use fresh, frozen, or even dried fruits.

The different fruits you can include are mango, pineapple, guava, pomegranate, kiwi, dragon fruit, apples, pears, plums, grapes, oranges, nectarines, bananas, watermelon, persimmon, mangosteen, lime, lemon, figs, apricots, prunes, peaches, honeydew melon, cantaloupe, jackfruit, lychees, cucumber, coconut, clementine, currants, durian, and grapefruit.

Berries are low in calories and rich in antioxidants and vitamins. There are various berries to choose from, like blackberries, blueberries, strawberries, goji berries, cranberries, mulberries, raspberries, and so on.

Starches are rich in complex carbs that supply your body with energy while filling up your tummy. Apart from this, they contain plenty of proteins, fibers, minerals, and amino acids. Whenever you are purchasing starches, stick to whole grains instead of the processed ones.

The different whole grains, you can include are rye, buckwheat, millet, quinoa, oats, wheat, wild rice, corn, barley, amaranth, whole wheat, bulgur, farro, kamut, millet, and einkorn. Apart from whole grains, you can also consume a variety of legumes. The different legumes you can start adding to your diet are pinto beans, black-eyed peas, black beans, chickpeas, fava beans, lentils, mung beans, navy beans, white beans, red beans, split peas, snow peas, sugar snap peas, soybeans, alfalfa sprouts, cannellini beans, azuki beans, lima beans, kidney beans, and green beans.

Herbs and spices not only help elevate the flavors of the food you consume but are also good for your health. Most of the herbs and spices tend to have anti-inflammatory properties. Regardless of whether you are using fresh or dried herbs, they are a great way to improve your overall health. While following a vegan diet, you can include all herbs and spices. For instance, you can add cilantro, bay leaf, star anise, basil, chamomile, celery, chili powder, chives, coriander, dill, garlic, ginger, lemongrass, nutmeg, nutritional yeast, onion powder, oregano, peppermint, pepper, parsley, mint, time, turmeric, saffron, rosemary, red pepper flakes, poppy seeds, and paprika.

All fats are not created equal. There are some unhealthy fats and some extremely healthy ones. Saturated fats and trans fats are undesirable and are the reasons why fats tend to get a bad rap.

However, the fats present in whole plant foods are extremely good for the overall functioning of your body. They enable the proper development as well as the functioning of the nervous system, improve the absorption of nutrients, and promote the heart's health. Including a variety of healthy, plant-based fats provides Linoleic acid and alpha-linolenic acids. Consuming sufficient healthy fats ensures that there exists a balance between omega-3 fatty acids and omega-6 fatty acids in your body. However, you need to be mindful of the fat consumption.

The different sources of healthy fats include nuts, seeds, and butter made from various nuts and seeds. You can start adding chia seeds, hemp seeds, flax seeds, sesame seeds, sunflower seeds, pumpkin seeds, cashews, pistachios, almonds, Brazil nuts, chestnuts, macadamia nuts, hazelnuts, walnuts, and pine nuts to your daily diet. Other sources of healthy fats include avocados, olives, and oils made from these ingredients.

The different condiments you can include are salsa, mustard, hummus, harissa, coconut milk, baked beans, applesauce, canned tomatoes, curry paste, guacamole, miso, sambal, vinegar, and tahini. Various vegan-friendly sweeteners, you can use include stevia, date syrup, coconut syrup, maple syrup, rice syrup, molasses, organic cane sugar, and agave syrup. Other miscellaneous ingredients include trail mix, coffee, cocoa, baking powder, cornstarch, tea, and potato starch.

# Chapter 6: Breakfast

## Tropi-Kale Breeze

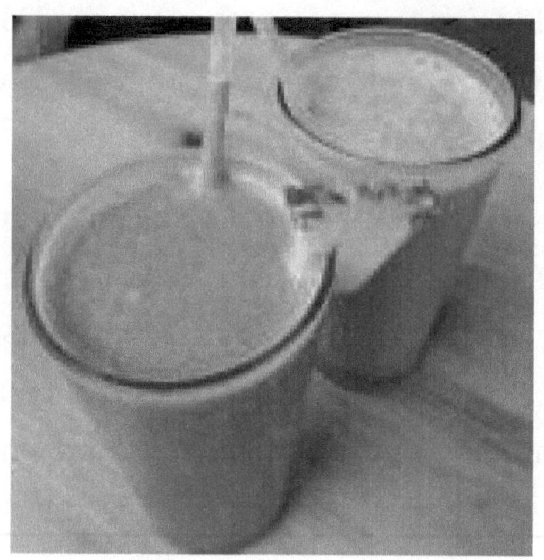

Preparation Time: 5 minutes

Cooking Time: ominutes

Servings: 4

Ingredients

1 cup chopped pineapple (frozen or fresh)

1 cup chopped mango (frozen or fresh)

½ to 1 cup chopped kale

½ avocado

½ cup coconut milk

1 cup water, or coconut water

1 teaspoon matcha green tea powder (optional)

Directions

Preparing the Ingredients.

Purée everything in a blender until smooth, adding more water (or coconut milk) if needed.

# Tofu-Spinach Scramble

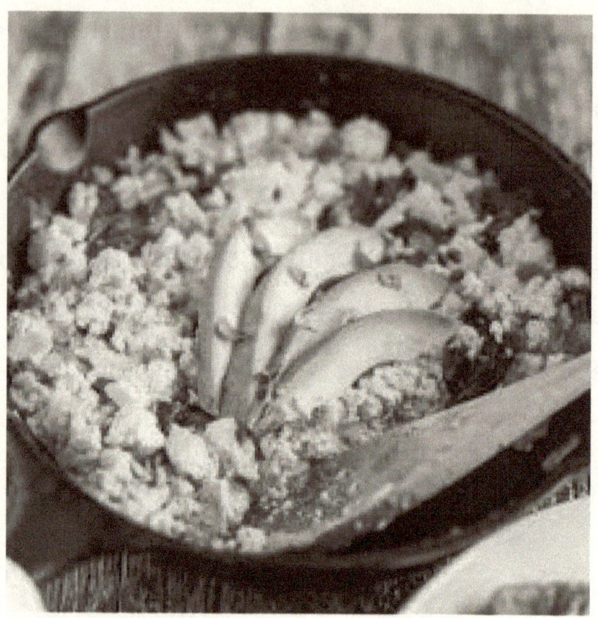

Preparation Time: 20 minutes

Cooking Time: 15 minutes

Servings: 5

Ingredients

1 (14-ounce) package water-packed extra-firm tofu

1 teaspoon extra-virgin olive oil or ¼ cup vegetable broth

1 small yellow onion, diced

3 teaspoons minced garlic (about 3 cloves)

3 large celery stalks, chopped

2 large carrots, peeled (optional) and chopped

1 teaspoon chili powder

½ teaspoon ground cumin

½ teaspoon ground turmeric

½ teaspoon salt (optional)

¼ teaspoon freshly ground black pepper

5 cups loosely packed spinach

Directions

Preparing the Ingredients.

Press and drain the tofu by placing it, wrapped in a paper towel, on a plate in the sink. Place a cutting board over the tofu, then set a heavy pot, can, or cookbook on the cutting board. Remove after 10 minutes. (Alternatively, use a tofu press.)

In a medium bowl, crumble the tofu with your hands or a potato masher. Set aside.

In a large skillet over medium-high heat, heat the olive oil. Add the onion, garlic, celery, and carrots, and sauté for 5 minutes, until the onion is softened.

Add the crumbled tofu, chili powder, cumin, turmeric, salt (if using), and pepper, and continue cooking for 7 to 8 more minutes, stirring frequently, until the tofu begins to brown.

Add the spinach and mix well. Cover and reduce the heat to medium. Steam the spinach for 3 minutes.

Divide evenly among 5 single-serving containers. Let cool before sealing the lids.

Place the airtight containers in the refrigerator for 5 days or freeze for up to 1 month. To thaw, refrigerate overnight. Reheat in the microwave for 2½ minutes or in a skillet over medium-high heat for 6 to 8 minutes.

# Chai Chia Smoothie

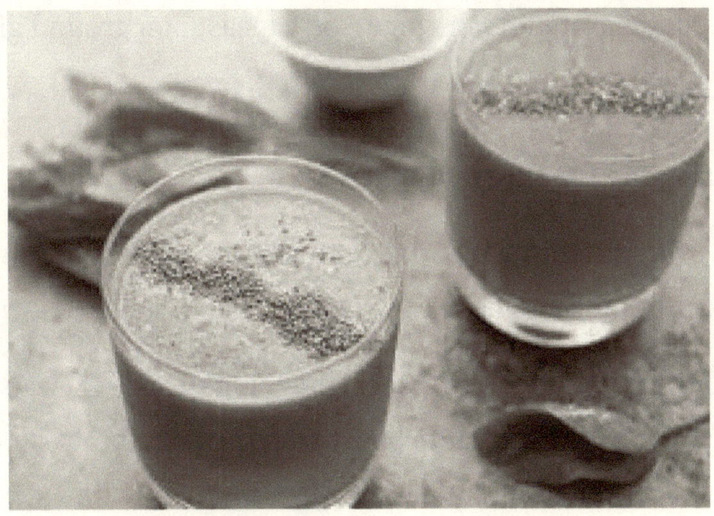

Preparation Time: 5 minutes

Cooking Time: 0minutes

Servings: 3

Ingredients

1 banana

½ cup coconut milk

1 cup water

1 cup alfalfa sprouts (optional)

1 to 2 soft Medjool dates, pitted

1 tablespoon chia seeds, or ground flax or hemp hearts

¼ teaspoon ground cinnamon

Pinch ground cardamom

1 tablespoon grated fresh ginger, or ¼ teaspoon ground ginger

Directions

Preparing the Ingredients.

Purée everything in a blender until smooth, adding more water (or coconut milk) if needed.

Although dates are super sweet, they don't cause a large blood sugar spike. They're great to boost sweetness while also boosting your intake of fiber and potassium.

# Banana Bread Rice Pudding

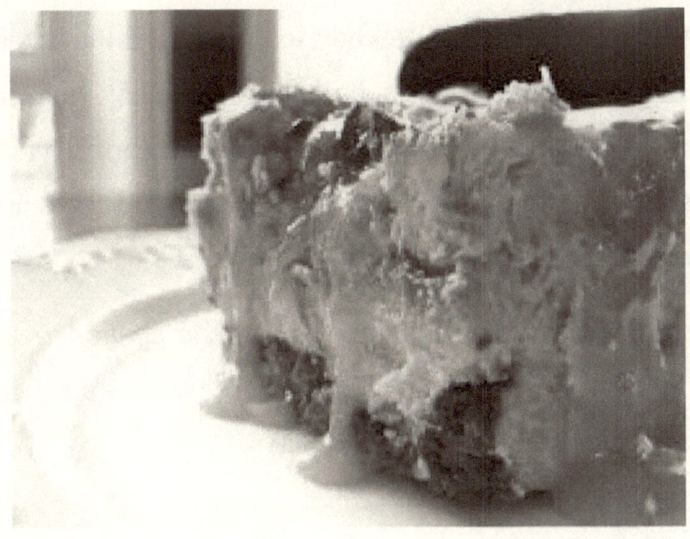

Preparation Time: 5 minutes

Servings: 4

Ingredients

1 cup rice

1½ cups water

1½ cups nondairy milk

3 tablespoons sugar (omit if using a sweetened nondairy milk)

2 teaspoons pumpkin pie spice or ground cinnamon

2 bananas

3 tablespoons chopped walnuts or sunflower seeds (optional)

Directions

Preparing the Ingredients.

In a medium pot, combine the rice, water, milk, sugar, and pumpkin pie spice. Bring to a boil over high heat, turn the heat to low, and cover the pot. Simmer, stirring occasionally, until the rice is soft and the liquid is absorbed. White rice takes about 20 minutes; brown rice takes about 50 minutes.

Smash the bananas and stir them into the cooked rice. Serve topped with walnuts (if using). Leftovers will keep refrigerated in an airtight container for up to 5 days.

# Broiled Grapefruit with Cinnamon Pitas

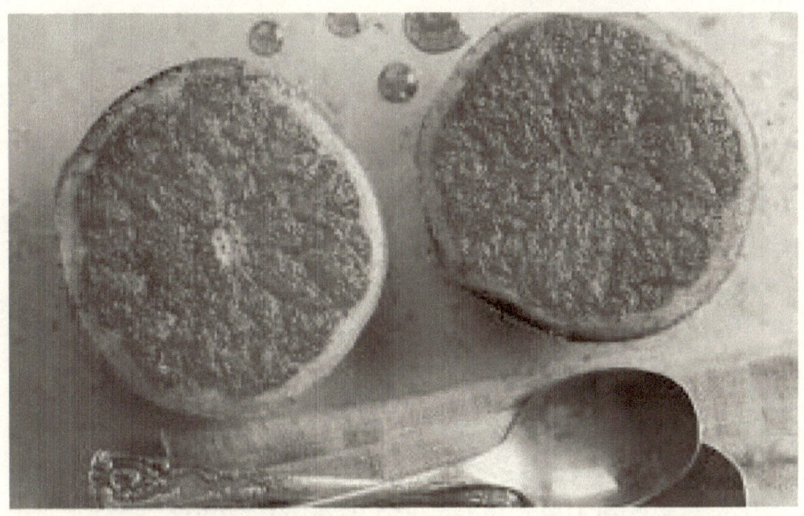

Preparation Time: 10 minutes

Cooking Time: 15 minutes

Servings: 5

Ingredients

2 whole-wheat pitas, cut into wedges

2 tablespoons coconut oil, melted

1 tablespoon ground cinnamon

2 tablespoons brown sugar

1 grapefruit, halved

2 tablespoons pure maple syrup or agave

Directions

Preparing the Ingredients.

Preheat the oven to 375°F.

Line a baking sheet with parchment paper.

Spread pita wedges in a single layer on a baking sheet and brush with melted coconut oil.

In a small bowl, combine the cinnamon and brown sugar and sprinkle over the pita wedges.

Bake in preheated oven until the wedges are crisp, about 8 minutes. Transfer the pita wedges to a plate and set aside.

Turn the oven to broil. Place the grapefruit halves on the baking sheet. Drizzle the maple syrup over the top of the grapefruit, if using. Broil until the syrup bubbles and begins to crystallize, 3 to 5 minutes. Serve immediately.

# Chocolate PB Smoothie

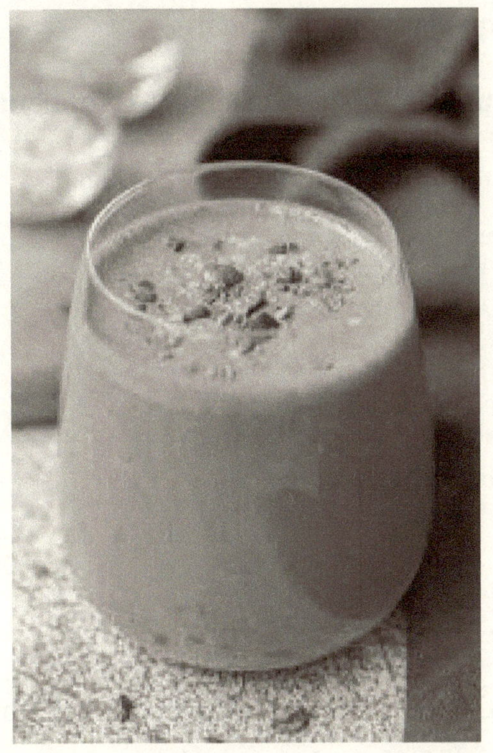

Preparation Time: 5 minutes

Cooking Time: 0 minutes

Servings: 4

Ingredients

1 banana

¼ cup rolled oats, or 1 scoop plan t protein powder

1 tablespoon flaxseed, or chia seeds

1 tablespoon unsweetened cocoa powder

1 tablespoon peanut butter, or almond or sunflower seed butter

1 tablespoon maple syrup (optional)

1 cup alfalfa sprouts, or spinach, chopped (optional)

½ cup nondairy milk (optional)

1 cup water

OPTIONAL

1 teaspoon maca powder

1 teaspoon cocoa nibs

Directions

Preparing the Ingredients.

Purée everything in a blender until smooth, adding more water (or nondairy milk) if needed. Add bonus boosters, as desired. Purée until blended.

# Orange French Toast

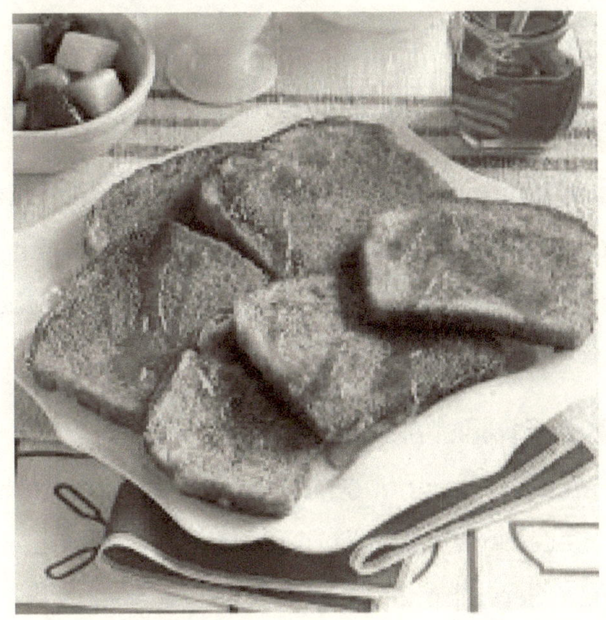

Preparation Time: 15 minutes

Cooking Time: 10 minutes

Servings: 4

Ingredients

3 very ripe bananas

1 cup unsweetened nondairy milk

zest and juice of 1 orange

1 teaspoon ground cinnamon

¼ teaspoon grated nutmeg

4 slices french bread

1 tablespoon coconut oil

Directions

Preparing the Ingredients.

In a blender, combine the bananas, almond milk, orange juice and zest, cinnamon, and nutmeg and blend until smooth. Pour the mixture into a 9-by-13-inch baking dish. Soak the bread in the mixture for 5 minutes on each side.

While the bread soaks, heat a griddle or sauté pan over medium-high heat. Melt the coconut oil in the pan and swirl to coat. Cook the bread slices until golden brown on both sides, about 5 minutes each. Serve immediately.

# Oatmeal Raisin Breakfast Cookie

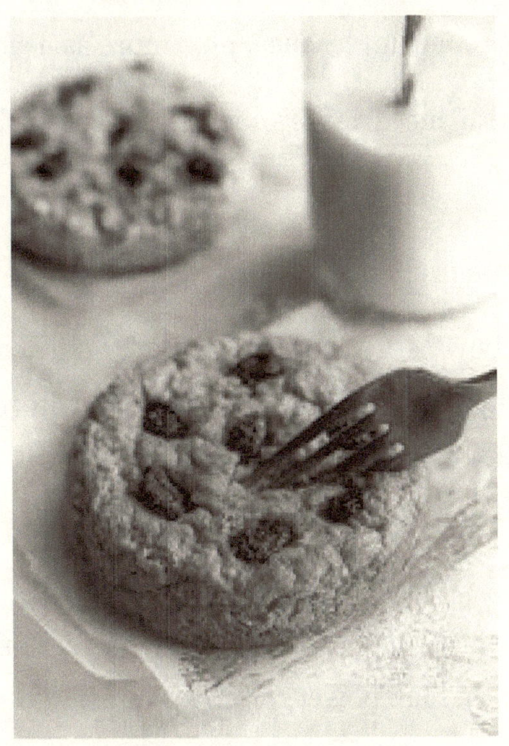

Preparation Time: 5 minutes

Cooking Time: 15 minutes

Servings: 2 cookies

Ingredients

½ cup rolled oats

1 tablespoon whole-wheat flour

½ teaspoon baking powder

1 to 2 tablespoons brown sugar

½ teaspoon pumpkin pie spice or ground cinnamon (optional)

¼ cup unsweetened applesauce, plus more as needed

2 tablespoons raisins, dried cranberries, or vegan chocolate chips

Directions

Preparing the Ingredients.

In a medium bowl, stir together the oats, flour, baking powder, sugar, and pumpkin pie spice (if using). Stir in the applesauce until thoroughly combined. Add another 1 to 2 tablespoons of applesauce if the mixture looks too dry (this will depend on the type of oats used).

Shape the mixture into 2 cookies. Put them on a microwave-safe plate and heat on high power for 90 seconds. Alternatively, bake on a small tray in a 350°F oven or toaster oven for 15 minutes. Let cool slightly before eating.

## Berry Beetsicle Smoothie

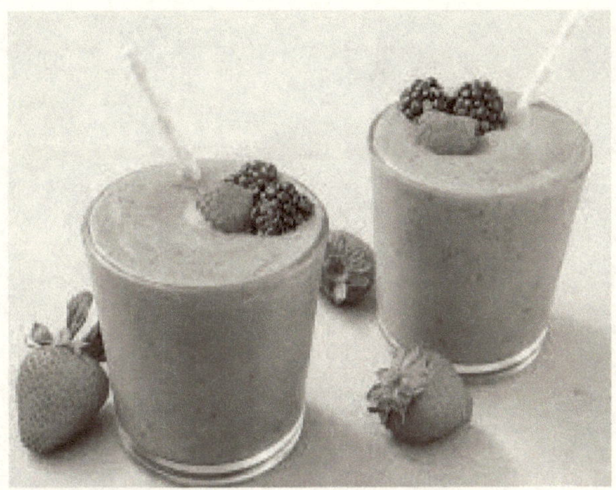

Preparation Time: 3 minutes

Cooking Time: 0minutes

Servings: 1

Ingredients

½ cup peeled and diced beets

½ cup frozen raspberries

1 frozen banana

1 tablespoon maple syrup

1 cup unsweetened soy or almond milk

Directions

Preparing the Ingredients.

Combine all the ingredients in a blender and blend until smooth.

# Blueberry Oat Muffins

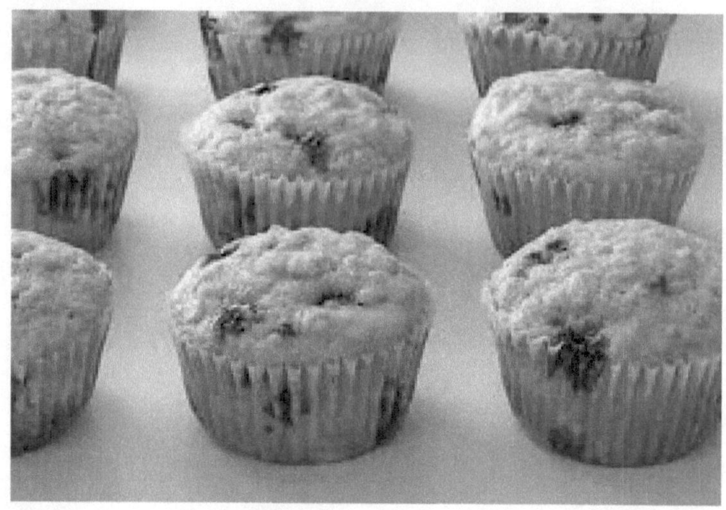

Preparation Time: 10 minutes

Cooking Time: 20 minutes

Servings: 12 mufins

Ingredients

2 tablespoons coconut oil or vegan margarine, melted, plus more for preparing the muffin tin

1 cup quick-cooking oats or instant oats

1 cup boiling water

½ cup nondairy milk

¼ cup ground flaxseed

1 teaspoon vanilla extract

1 teaspoon apple cider vinegar

1½ cups whole-wheat flour

½ cup brown sugar

2 teaspoons baking soda

Pinch salt

1 cup blueberries

Directions

Preparing the Ingredients.

Preheat the oven to 400°F.

Coat a muffin tin with coconut oil, line with paper muffin cups, or use a nonstick tin.

In a large bowl, combine the oats and boiling water. Stir so the oats soften. Add the coconut oil, milk, flaxseed, vanilla, and vinegar and stir to combine. Add the flour, sugar, baking soda, and salt. Stir until just combined. Gently fold in the blueberries. Scoop the muffin mixture into the prepared tin, about ⅓ cup for each muffin.

Bake for 20 to 25 minutes, until slightly browned on top and springy to the touch. Let cool for about 10 minutes. Run a dinner knife around the inside of each cup to loosen, then tilt the muffins on their sides in the muffin wells so air gets underneath. These keep in an airtight container in the refrigerator for up to 1 week or in the freezer indefinitely.

# Quinoa Applesauce Muffins

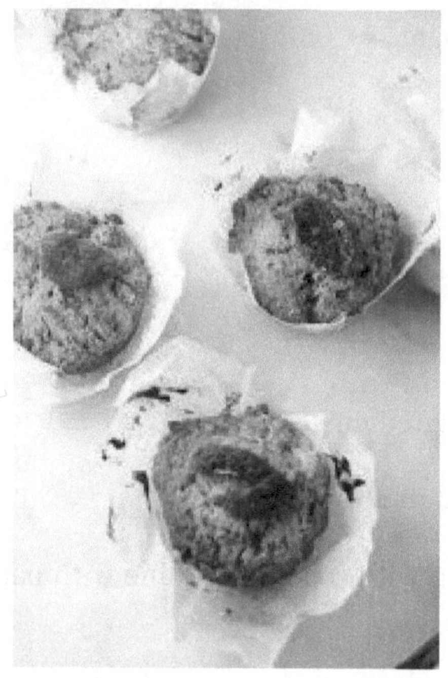

Preparation Time: 10 minutes

Cooking Time: 15 minutes

Servings: 5

Ingredients

2 tablespoons coconut oil or margarine, melted, plus more for coating the muffin tin

¼ cup ground flaxseed

½ cup water

2 cups unsweetened applesauce

½ cup brown sugar

1 teaspoon apple cider vinegar

2½ cups whole-wheat flour

1½ cups cooked quinoa

2 teaspoons baking soda

Pinch salt

½ cup dried cranberries or raisins

Directions

Preparing the Ingredients.

Preheat the oven to 400°F.

Coat a muffin tin with coconut oil, line with paper muffin cups, or use a nonstick tin. In a large bowl, stir together the flaxseed and water. Add the applesauce, sugar, coconut oil, and vinegar. Stir to combine. Add the flour, quinoa, baking soda, and salt, stirring until just combined. Gently fold in the cranberries without stirring too much. Scoop the muffin mixture into the prepared tin, about ⅓ cup for each muffin.

Bake for 15 to 20 minutes, until slightly browned on top and springy to the touch. Let cool for about 10 minutes. Run a dinner knife around the inside of each cup to loosen, then tilt the muffins on their sides in the muffin wells so air gets underneath. These keep in an airtight container in the refrigerator for up to 1 week or in the freezer indefinitely.

# Pumpkin Pancakes

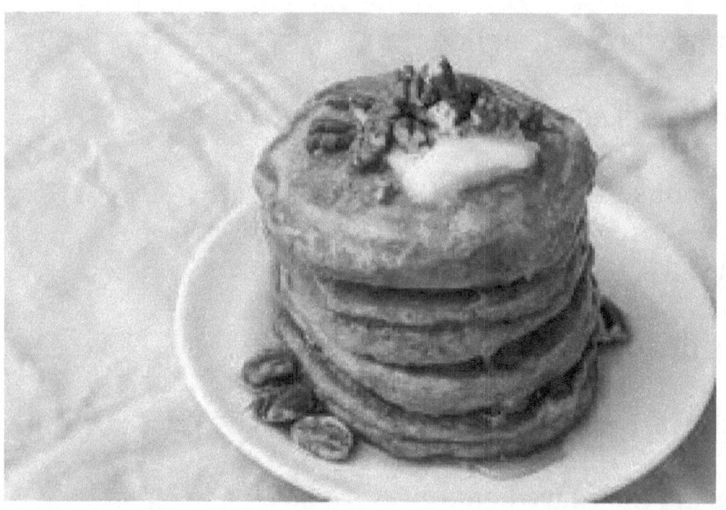

Preparation Time: 15 minutes

Cooking Time: 15 minutes

Servings: 4

Ingredients

2 cups unsweetened almond milk

1 teaspoon apple cider vinegar

2½ cups whole-wheat flour

2 tablespoons baking powder

½ teaspoon baking soda

1 teaspoon sea salt

1 teaspoon pumpkin pie spice or ½ teaspoon ground cinnamon plus ¼ teaspoon grated nutmeg plus ¼ teaspoon ground allspice

½ cup canned pumpkin purée

1 cup water

1 tablespoon coconut oil

Directions

Preparing the Ingredients.

In a small bowl, combine the almond milk and apple cider vinegar. Set aside.

In a large bowl, whisk together the flour, baking powder, baking soda, salt, and pumpkin pie spice. In another large bowl, combine the almond milk mixture, pumpkin purée, and water, whisking to mix well. Add the wet ingredients to the dry ingredients and fold together until the dry ingredients are just moistened. You will still have a few streaks of flour in the bowl.

In a nonstick pan or griddle over medium-high heat, melt the coconut oil and swirl to coat. Pour the batter into the pan ¼ cup at a time and cook until the pancakes are browned, about 5 minutes per side. Serve immediately.

# Green Breakfast Smoothie

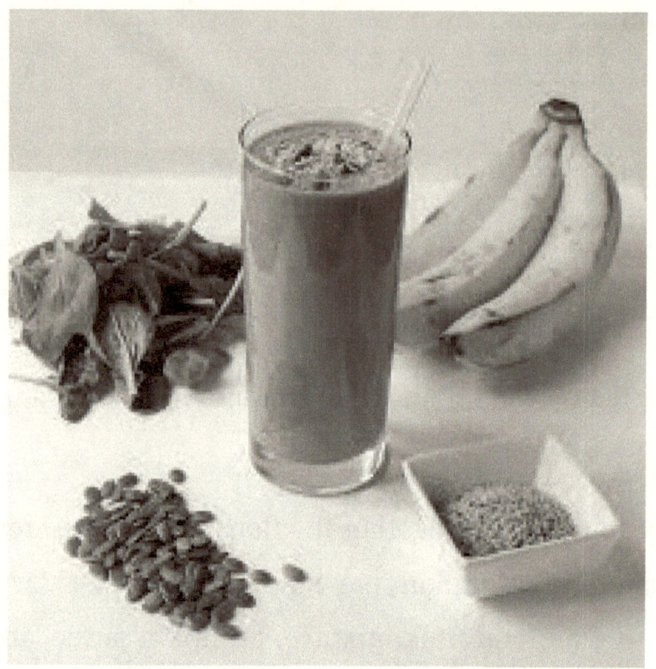

Preparation Time: 10 minutes

Cooking Time: 0 minutes

Servings: 2

Ingredients

½ banana, sliced

2 Cups Spinach or other greens, such as kale

1 Cup sliced berries of your choosing, fresh or frozen

1 orange, peeled and cut into segments

1 cup unsweetened nondairy milk

1 cup ice

Directions

Preparing the Ingredients. In a blender, combine all the ingredients.

Starting with the blender on low speed, begin blending the smoothie, gradually increasing blender speed until smooth. Serve immediately.

# Blueberry Lemonade Smoothie

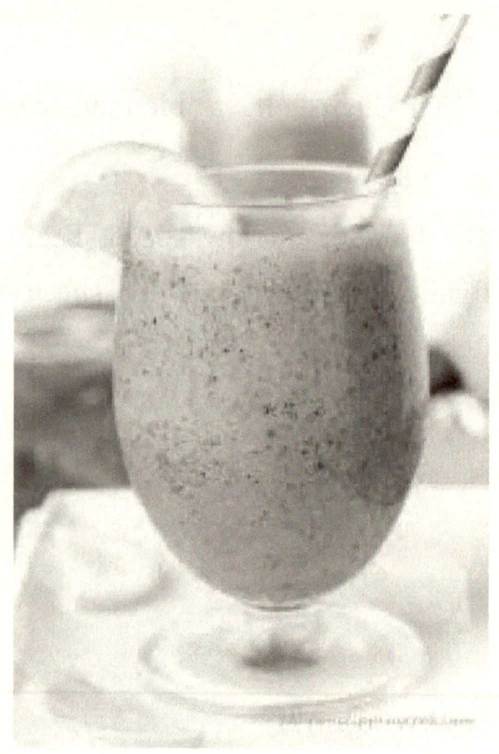

Preparation Time: 5 minutes

Cooking Time: 0 minutes

Servings: 1

Ingredients

1 cup roughly chopped kale

¾ cup frozen blueberries

1 cup unsweetened soy or almond milk

Juice of 1 lemon

1 tablespoon maple syrup

Directions

Preparing the Ingredients.

Combine all the ingredients in a blender and blend until smooth. Enjoy immediately.

# Berry Protein Smoothie

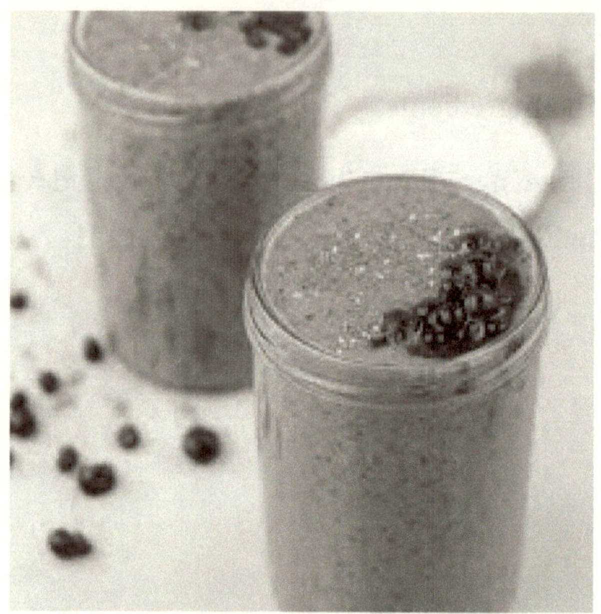

Preparation Time: 5 minutes

Cooking Time: 0 minutes

Servings: 1

Ingredients

1 banana

1 cup fresh or frozen berries

¾ cup water or nondairy milk, plus more as needed

1 scoop plant-based protein powder, 3 ounces silken tofu, ¼ cup rolled oats, or ½ cup cooked quinoa

Additions

1 tablespoon ground flaxseed or chia seeds

1 handful fresh spinach or lettuce, or 1 chunk cucumber

coconut water to replace some of the liquid

Directions

Preparing the Ingredients

In a blender, combine the banana, berries, water, and your choice of protein.

Add any addition ingredients as desired. Purée until smooth and creamy, about 50 seconds.

Add a bit more water if you like a thinner smoothie.

# Flaxseed Porridge

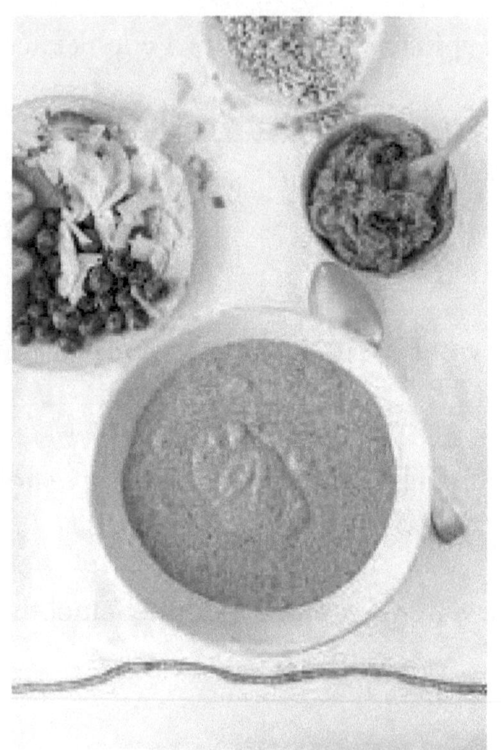

Servings: 2

Preparation Time: 15 Minutes

Ingredients:

1 Cup Almond Milk

1 Teaspoon Cinnamon

¼ Cup Coconut Flour

¼ Cup Ground Flaxseed

10 Drops Stevia

1 Teaspoon Vanilla Extract, Pure

Pinch Sea Salt

1 Ounces Coconut, Shaved for Garnish

2 Ounces Blueberries for Garnish

2 Tablespoons Almond Butter for Garnish

2 Tablespoons Pumpkin Seeds for Garnish

Directions:

Heat your almond milk in a saucepan using low heat, and whisk your coconut flour, salt, cinnamon and flaxseed together.

Add in your stevia and vanilla once it's bubbling

Remove it from heat, mixing all of your ingredients together.

Garnish with blueberries, coconut, pumpkin seeds and almonds before serving.

# Spicy Hash Browns

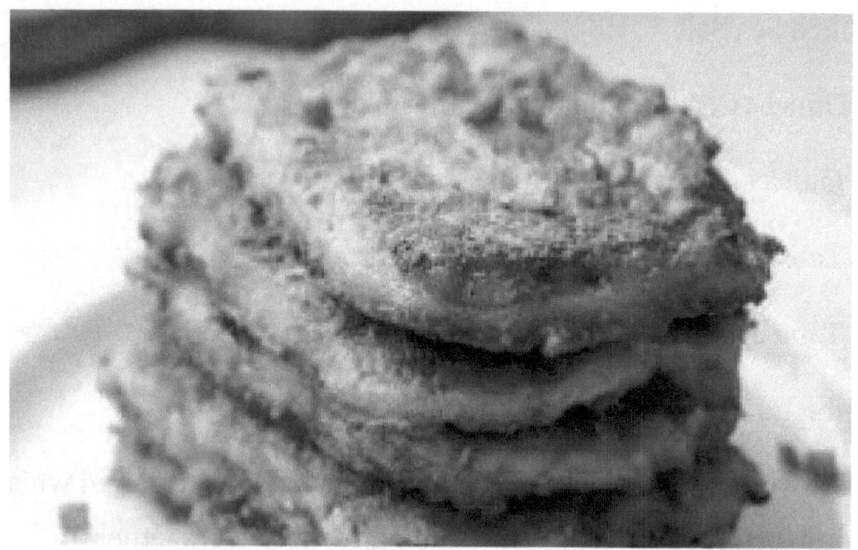

Preparation Time: 15 Minutes

Servings: 5

Ingredients:

1 Teaspoon Paprika

¼ Teaspoon Red Pepper

¾ Teaspoon Chili Powder

2 Tablespoons Olive Oil

6 ½ Cups Potatoes, Diced

Sea Salt & Black Pepper to Taste

Directions:

Start by heating you oven to 400, and then get out a large bowl.

Mix together your olive oil, chili powder, red peppers, salt, black pepper, and paprika. Stir well.

Coat your potatoes in the mixture, and then arrange your potatoes on a baking sheet in a single layer

Bake for about thirty minutes.

# Kiwi Slushie

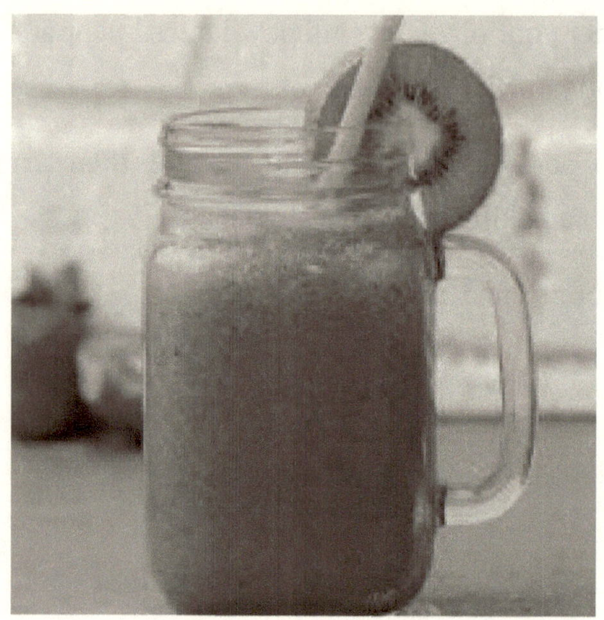

Servings: 2

Preparation Time: 5 Minutes

Ingredients:

18 Chocolate Tea Ice Cubes

1 Cup Vanilla Rice Milk

2 Ripe Kiwi Fruits, Sliced & Frozen

Directions:

Blend everything together until smooth.

# Chia Seed Smoothie

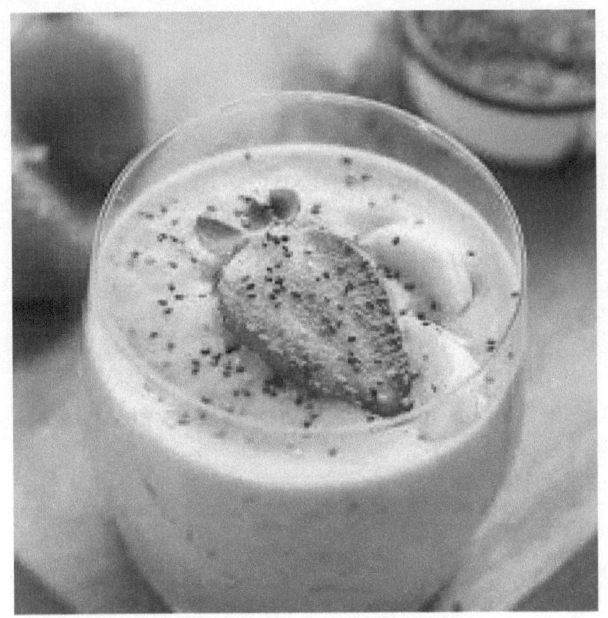

Servings: 3

Preparation Time: 5 Minutes

Ingredients:

¼ Teaspoon Cinnamon

1 Tablespoon Ginger, Fresh & Grated

Pinch Cardamom

1 Tablespoon Chia Seeds

2 Medjool Dates, Pitted

1 Cup Alfalfa Sprouts

1 Cup Water

1 Banana

½ Cup Coconut Milk, Unsweetened

Directions:

Blend everything together until smooth.

# Mango Smoothie

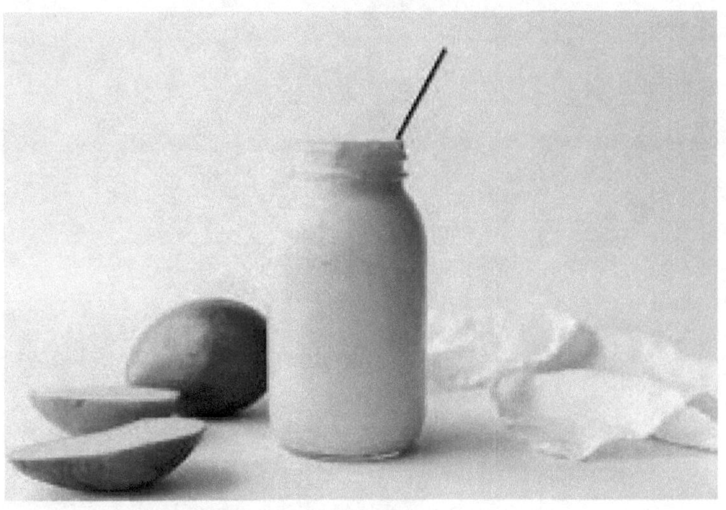

Servings: 3

Preparation Time: 5 Minutes

Ingredients:

1 Carrot, Peeled & Chopped

1 Cup Strawberries

1 Cup Water

1 Cup Peaches, Chopped

1 Banana, Frozen & sliced

1 Cup Mango, Chopped

Directions:

Blend everything together until smooth.

# Quinoa & Chocolate Bowl

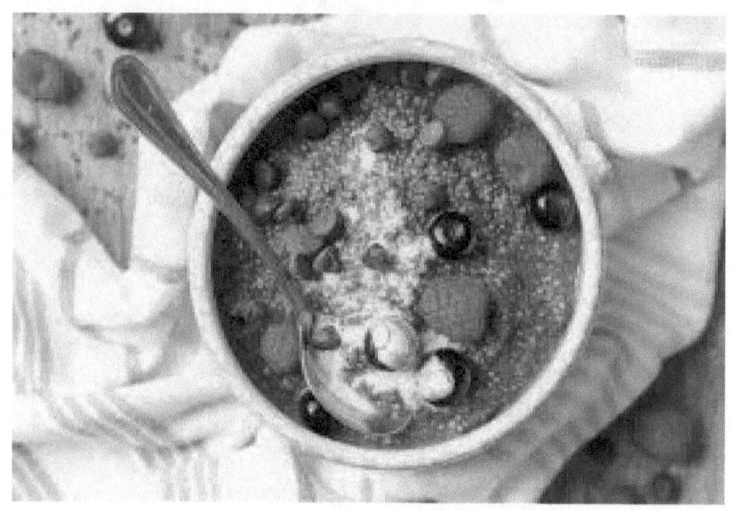

Servings: 2

Preparation Time: 35 Minutes

Ingredients:

1 Cup Quinoa

1 Cup Almond Milk, Unsweetened

1 Teaspoon Cinnamon

1 Banana

1 Cup Water

2-3 Tablespoons Cocoa Powder, Unsweetened

2 Tablespoons Almond Butter

1 Tablespoon Chia Seeds, Ground

2 Tablespoons Walnuts, Optional

¼ Cup Raspberries, Fresh

Directions:

Place your cinnamon, milk, water and quinoa in a pot, bringing it to a boil before turning it down to low heat to simmer. Cover, simmering for twenty-five to thirty minutes.

Puree your banana, mixing in your almond butter, flaxseed and cocoa powder.

Scoop a cup of quinoa into a bowl, and then top with pudding, raspberries and walnuts if you're using them before serving.

# Vegetable Hash

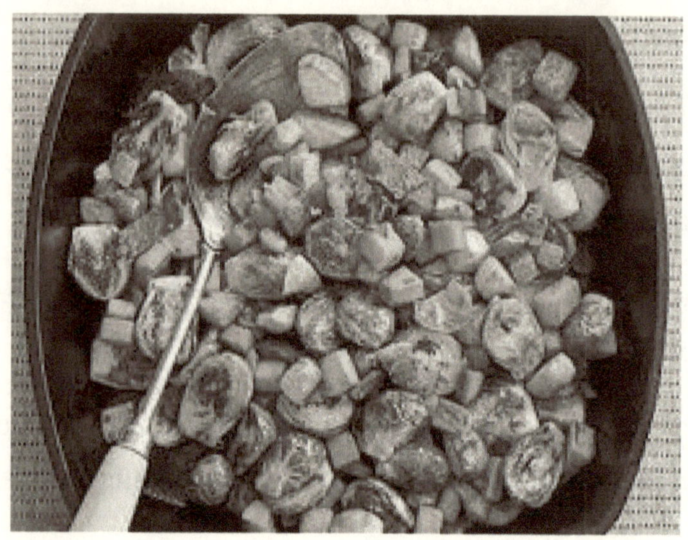

Servings: 4

Preparation Time: 35 Minutes

Ingredients:

1 Tablespoon Sage Leaves, Chopped

1 Bell Pepper, Diced

3 Cloves Garlic, Minced

1 Onion, Diced

3 Tablespoons Olive Oil

3 Red Potatoes, Diced

15 Ounces Black Beans, Canned

1 Tablespoon Parsley, Chopped

2 Cups Swiss Chard, Chopped

Sea Salt & Black Pepper to Taste

Directions:

Start by cooking your potato, garlic and onion in a skillet with your oil. This will take twenty minutes.

Add in your Swiss chard and beans, cooking for three more minutes.

Season with salt and pepper, and serve with parsley.

# Walnut Porridge

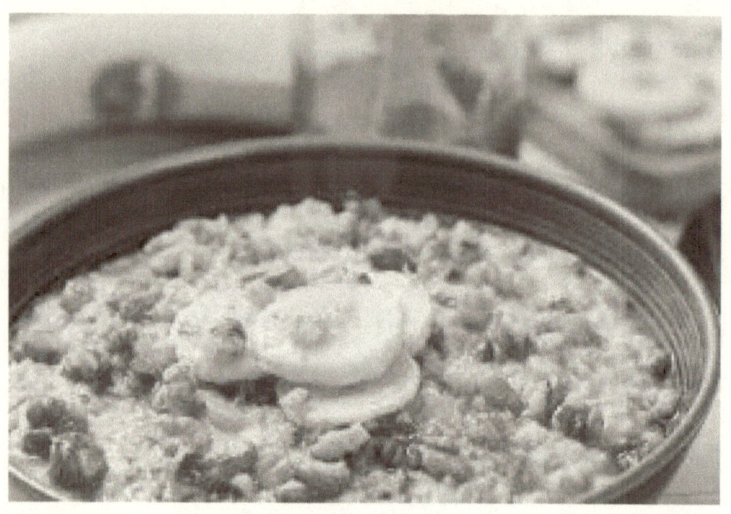

Servings: 2

Preparation Time: 25 Minutes

Ingredients:

1 ½ Cups Water

½ Cup Coconut Milk, Unsweetened

1 Cup Teff, Whole Grain

½ Teaspoon Cardamom, Ground

1 Teaspoon Sea Salt, Fine

¼ Cup Walnuts, Chopped

1 Tablespoon Maple Syrup, Pure

Directions:

Start by combining your coconut oil and water, bringing it to a boil before stirring in your teff.

Add the cardamom, and then allow it to simmer for twenty minutes.

Mix in your walnuts and maple syrup before serving.

# Granola

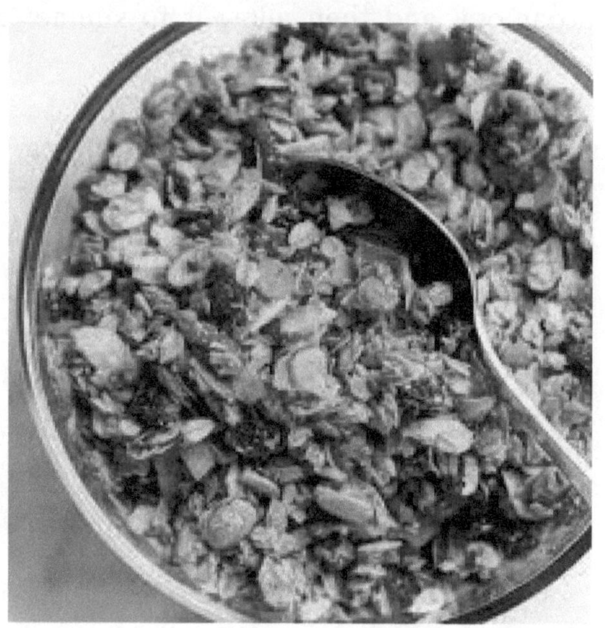

Servings: 7

Preparation Time: 1 Hour 30 Minutes

Ingredients:

½ Cup Maple Syrup , Pure

¼ Cup Coconut Oil

¾ Cup Coconut, Unsweetened & Shredded

1 Cup Almonds, Slivered

¾ Teaspoon Sea Salt, Fine

5 Cups Rolled Oats

Directions:

Start by heating your oven to 250, and then mix all of your ingredients together in a bowl.

Spread your granola out over two baking sheets, making sure it's spread out evenly.

Bake for an hour and fifteen minutes, but you'll need to stir every twenty minutes.

Allow it to cool before serving.

# Breakfast Cereal

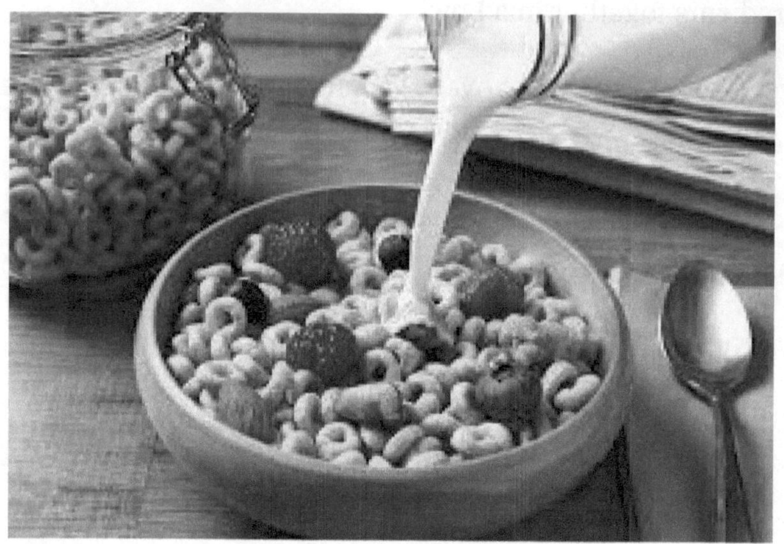

Servings: 6

Preparation Time: 45 Minutes

Ingredients:

¼ Tablespoon Butter

2 ¼ Cups Water

Honey to Taste

1 Teaspoon Cinnamon

1 Cup Brown Rice, Uncooked

½ Cup Raisins, Seedless

Directions:

Start by combining your cinnamon, raisins, rice, and butter in a saucepan before adding in your water. Bring it to a boil, and allow it to simmer while covered for forty minutes. Fluff with a fork.

Serve with honey.

# Fruity Oatmeal

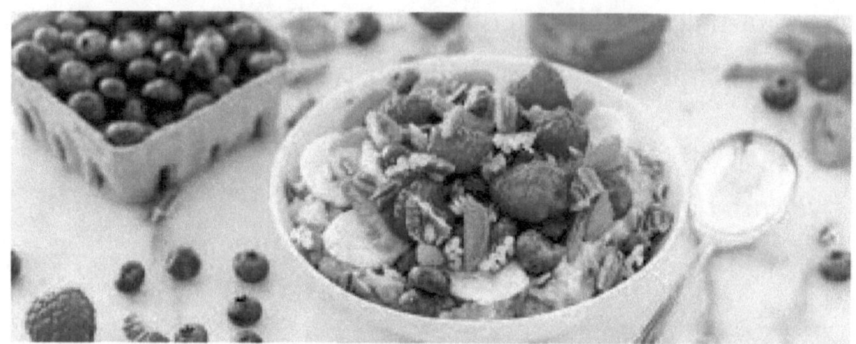

Servings: 2

Preparation Time: 20 minutes

Cooking Time: 15 minutes

Servings: 5

Ingredients:

½ Cup Apple Juice, Fresh & Frozen

½ Cup Oatmeal

½ Cup Water

3 Prunes, Diced

1 Apple, Small & Diced

4 Pecans, Diced

3 Apricots, Dehydrated, Dried & Diced

¼ Teaspoon Cinnamon

Directions:

Start by getting out a small saucepan and mix together your apple juice and water, bringing the mixture to a boil.

Add a half a cup of oatmeal, cooking for a minute. Add in your pecans, cinnamon and fruit pieces. Make sure to stir. If you want to make sure you have more vitamins, add in your fruit when your oatmeal is nearly cool.

# Pecan Pumpkin Spice Oatmeal

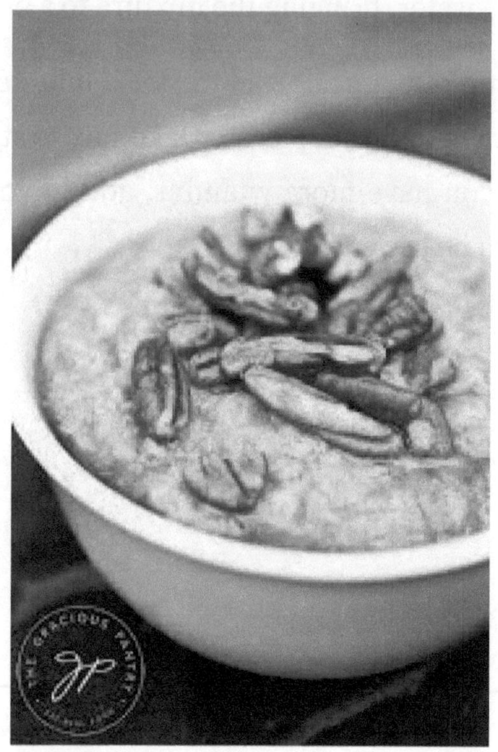

Cooking Time: 15 minutes

Servings: 5

Ingredients:

1/2 cup steel-cut oats

1/2 cup pumpkin purée

1 1/2 cups unsweetened almond milk

1/2 teaspoon cinnamon

1/8 teaspoon nutmeg

1 teaspoon vanilla extract

1/8 teaspoon of ground cloves

1/8 teaspoon ginger

1/4 cup brown sugar

Chopped pecans, for serving

Directions:

Spray the instant pot with nonstick spray. Combine everything except for the brown sugar and pecans.

Seal the lid and cook on high 3 minutes, then let the pressure release naturally.

Stir in the brown sugar and top with chopped pecans.

# Carrot Cake Oatmeal with Cream Cheese Frosting

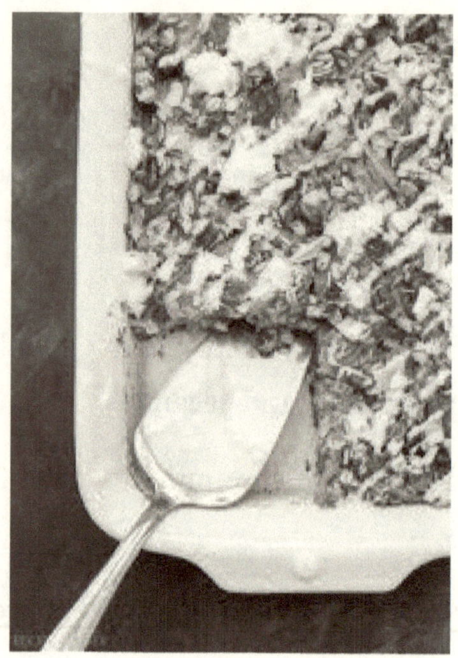

Cooking Time: 15 minutes

Servings: 5

Ingredients:

1 small white sweet potato, peeled and steamed

1 small carrot, grated

1/4 small zucchini, grated

1/2 cup steel-cut oats

1 1/2 cups nondairy milk

1/2 teaspoon lemon juice

1/2 teaspoon apple cider vinegar

1/8 teaspoon of salt

1/8 teaspoon ground cloves

1/8 teaspoon nutmeg

1/2 teaspoon cinnamon

2 tablespoons brown sugar

2 tablespoons maple syrup

1 1/2 tablespoons coconut oil

1 tablespoon water

Directions:

To make the cream cheese frosting, puree half of the steamed sweet potato in a food processor. Add the maple syrup, water, coconut oil, lemon juice, and apple cider vinegar and puree until smooth. Add more sweet potato if the mixture is not thick enough.

Spray the instant pot with nonstick spray. Combine the rest of the ingredients, then seal the lid and cook on high 3 minutes.

Let the pressure release naturally. Add additional milk to the oatmeal if needed, and top each serving with a dollop of the cream cheese frosting.

# Chocolate Walnut Oatmeal

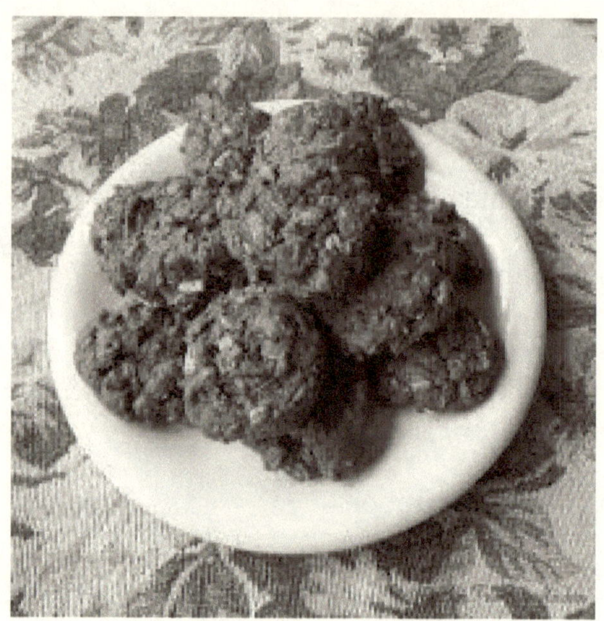

Preparation Time: 20 minutes

Cooking Time: 15 minutes

Servings: 5

Ingredients:

1/2 cup steel-cut oats

2 tablespoons cocoa powder

1 teaspoon brown sugar

1 tablespoon agave nectar

1 teaspoon vanilla extract

1/2 cup unsweetened almond milk

1 1/2 cups water

Semisweet chocolate chips, for topping

Walnuts for topping

Directions:

Spray the instant pot with nonstick spray. Combine the oats, cocoa powder, water, vanilla, brown sugar, and agave nectar.

Cook on high 3 minutes, then let the pressure release naturally. Stir in the almond milk.

Top with chocolate chips and walnuts.

# Breakfast Burrito Filling

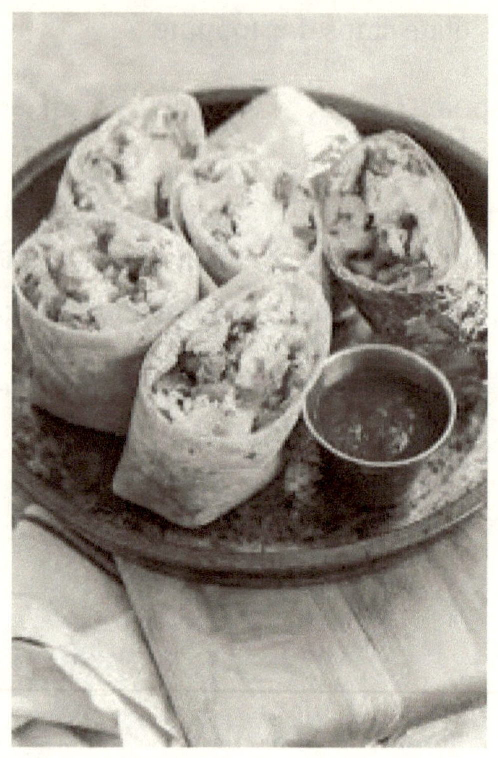

Preparation Time: 20 minutes

Cooking Time: 15 minutes

Servings: 2

Ingredients:

15 ounces tofu, drained and crumbled

1/2 cup water

1 clove garlic, minced

1/2 bell pepper, chopped

1/2 teaspoon chili powder

1/4 teaspoon chipotle chili powder

1/4 teaspoon sriracha sauce

1 teaspoon lime juice

Salt and pepper, to taste

1/4 cup shredded vegan cheddar cheese, for serving

Warm tortillas, for serving

Salsa, for serving

Directions:

Combine all the ingredients in the instant pot. Seal the lid and cook on high 4 minutes, then let the pressure release naturally.

If the mixture is too wet, drain off some of the water. Stir in the cheese to melt it. Serve wrapped warm tortillas with salsa.

# Tofu Breakfast Custard and Potatoes

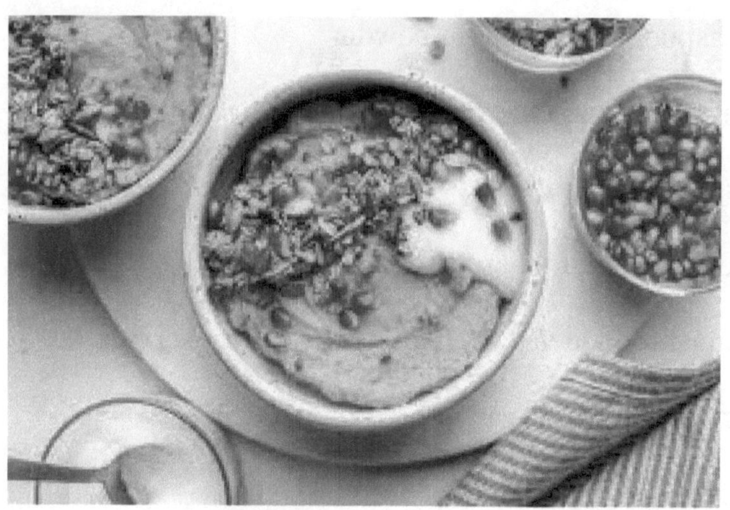

Preparation Time: 20 minutes

Cooking Time: 15 minutes

Servings: 2

Ingredients:

12 ounces frozen hash brow ns

1 shallot, chopped

2 tablespoons vegan chicken-flavored bouillon

10 ounces silken tofu

1/2 cup shredded vegan cheddar cheese

1/2 cup nondairy milk

1/4 teaspoon onion powder

1/8 teaspoon garlic powder

1/2 teaspoon seasoned salt

1/4 teaspoon freshly ground pepper

1 tablespoon olive oil

Hot sauce, for serving

Directions:

Puree the tofu, milk, bouillon, garlic powder, onion powder and seasoned salt in a food processor.

Heat the oil in the instant pot on the sauté setting and cook the shallot for 3 minutes.

Spread the hash browns on top of the cooked shallots, and top with the cheese. Pour the tofu puree over the top, then sprinkle with fresh ground pepper.

Cook on high 5 minutes, then quick release the pressure.

The tofu mixture should be a jiggly custard texture. If it is too moist, return the instant pot to the sauté setting and cook longer with the lid on but vented.

Serve with hot sauce!

# Apple and Sausage French Toast Casserole

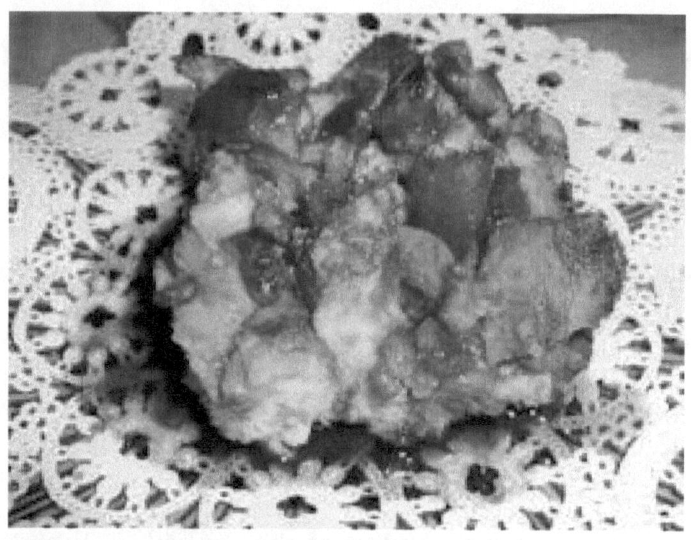

Preparation Time: 20 minutes

Cooking Time: 55 minutes

Servings: 2

Ingredients:

4 links vegan breakfast sausages, chopped into coins

2 apples, peeled and chopped

Juice of 1/2 lemon

Zest of 1/2 lemon

1/2 loaf whole wheat bread, chopped into cubes

1 1/2 cups water

1 teaspoon vanilla extract

3 tablespoons unsweetened applesauce

1/2 teaspoon cinnamon

1 tablespoon olive oil

Maple syrup, for serving

Directions:

Heat olive oil in the instant pot using the sauté setting. Add the sausage and cook for 10 minutes.

Add the water, applesauce, vanilla extract, lemon juice, and cinnamon to the instant pot. Add the apples, then the bread cubes. Push the bread down to make sure it is all coated with the mixture.

Seal the lid and cook on high 4 minutes, then let the pressure release naturally. Dust with powdered sugar and lemon zest and serve.

# **Granola.**

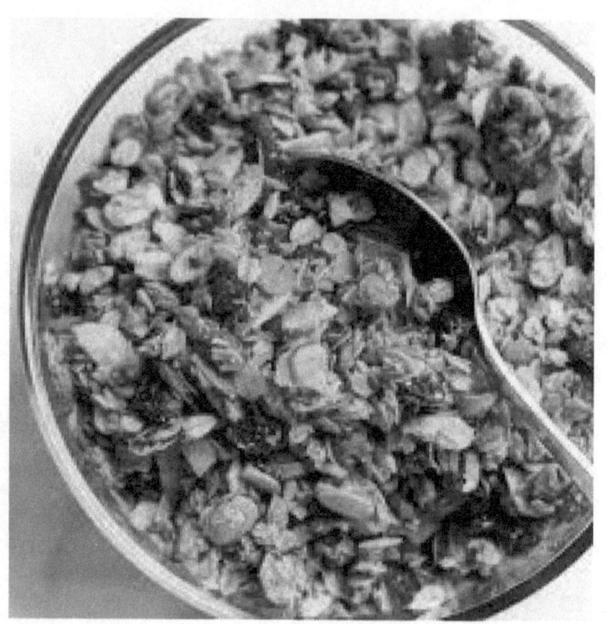

Preparation Time: 20 minutes

Cooking Time: 45 minutes

Servings: 2

Ingredients:

5 cups old-fashioned rolled oats

1 cup slivere d blanched almonds

⅔ cup pure maple syrup

½ cup wheat germ

½ cup unsweetened shredded coconut

½ cup sunflower seeds

½ cup golden raisins or sweetened dried cranberries

½ cup chopped dates or dried apricots

¼ cup vegetable oil

¼ cup packed light brown sugar

3 tablespoons water

1 teaspoon pure vanilla extract

Directions:

Spray the Instant Pot insert with cooking spray and set to high.

Add the maple syrup, oil, water, sugar, and vanilla.

In a bowl combine the oats, wheat germ, almonds, sunflower seeds, coconut, and dates.

Mix the oats into the syrup mix in the Instant Pot.

Seal and cook on Meat for 12 minutes.

Release the pressure and cook with the lid open until your granola is crisp.

# Chapter 7: Lunch

## Banh Mi

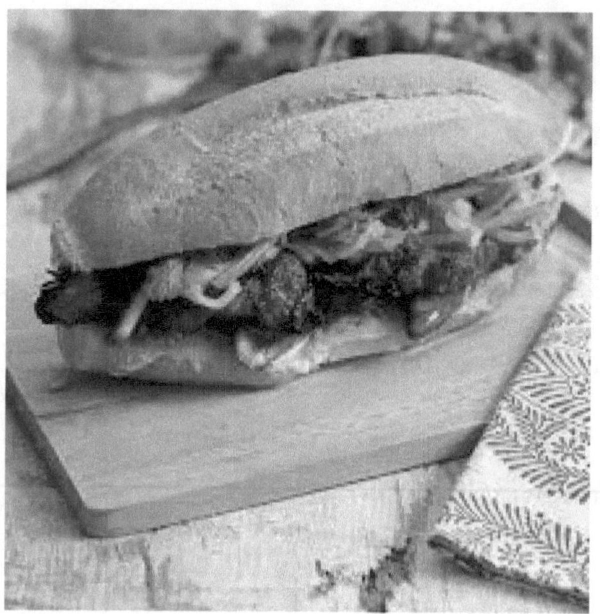

Cooking Time: 20 minutes

Servings: 4

Ingredients

1 ½ cup raw vegetables, cabbage and carrots, shredded

1 cup hummus

8 oz. cooked tempeh, very finely sliced

1 long French baguette

½ small pack coriander leaves

½ small pack mint leaves

3 tablespoons white wine vinegar

1 teaspoon golden caster sugar

hot sauce

salt, to taste

Instructions

Place vegetables, vinegar, caster sugar and salt in a large bowl, mix well and set aside to marinate.

Heat the oven to 360F.

Place baguette in the oven pan, slice it in 4 slices, and cook in the oven for 5 minutes.

Once done, remove from the oven, spread hummus on 2 slices, top with 4 tempeh pieces and pickled vegetables.

Sprinkle coriander, mint leaves and top with the other 2 remaining baguette slices.

# Sweet Potato Buddha Bowl Almond Butter Dressing

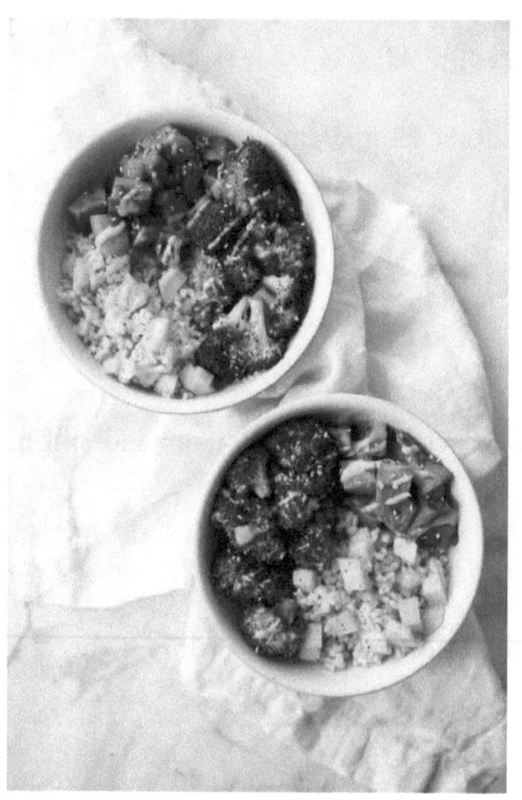

Cooking Time: 1 hour

Servings: 4

Ingredients

For the roasted vegetables:

1 large head broccoli, cut into florets

2 sweet potatoes, cubed

2 cloves garlic, minced

1 tablespoon toasted sesame oil

salt and pepper

For the mango coconut rice:

2 teaspoons coconut oil

1 cup unsweetened coconut milk

1 cup water

1 cup brown rice, uncooked

1 ripe mango, diced

For the almond butter dressing:

¼ cup natural creamy almond butter

4 tablespoons fresh orange juice

2 teaspoons maple syrup

½ teaspoon apple cider vinegar

1 teaspoon coconut oil, melted

Instructions

Place the pot over medium heat, add coconut oil.

Add brown rice and cook for 5 minutes, add water and coconut milk and bring it to a boil. Cover, reduce the heat and let it simmer for about 45 minutes.

When done add mango, salt, and set aside

Preheat the oven 375F and line a baking sheet with parchment paper.

Place sweet potatoes in a microwave safe bowl and heat it for about 4 minutes, then transfer to the prepared baking sheet.

Add broccoli florets, minced garlic to the baking sheet and mix well.

Bake in the oven for 30 minutes until tender.

Mix almond butter dressing ingredients in a medium bowl.

Serve rice in bowls, top with roasted vegetables and 2 tablespoons of the almond dressing.

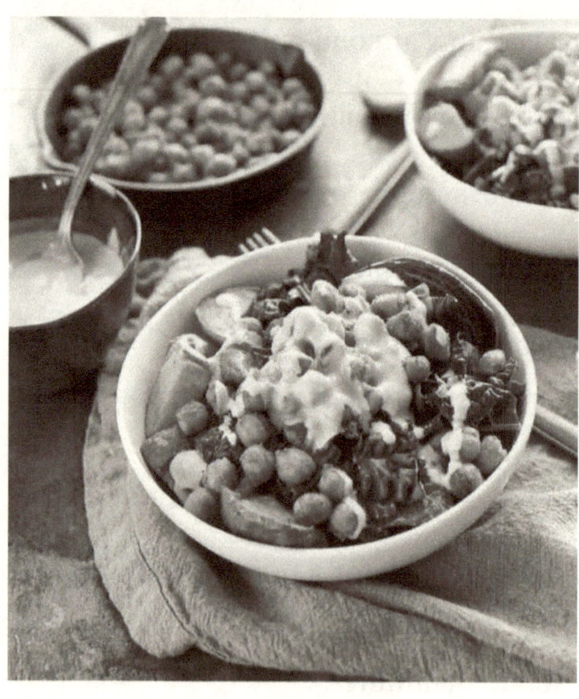

## Curry Spiced Sweet Potato Wild Rice Burgers

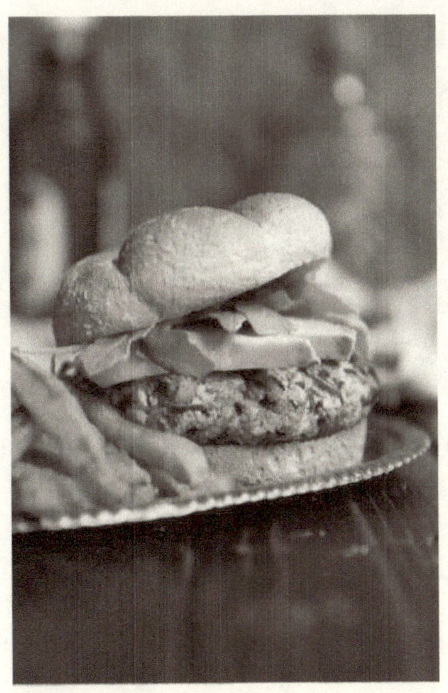

Cooking Time: 1 hour 15 minutes

Servings: 6

Ingredients

1 sweet potato

½ cup wild rice blend, uncooked

15 oz. can chickpeas, rinsed and drained

½ cup breadcrumbs

1/3 cup dried cranberries

2 teaspoons coconut oil

1 teaspoon curry powder

1 ½ teaspoons cumin

¼ teaspoon garlic powder

salt and pepper

Instructions

Prepare a pan with parchment lined paper and preheat the oven to 400F.

Place sweet potato on the pan and poke it with a fork. Bake for 45 minutes.

Place a small pan over medium heat. Add rice, water and bring to a boil. Cover, reduce the heat and let it simmer for 40 minutes.

Place sweet potato and chickpeas in a food processor, process for about 10 seconds and transfer to a large bowl.

Add cooked rice, curry powder, cumin, garlic, salt, pepper and mix well.

Add breadcrumbs, cranberries, pecans, mix well and scoop the mixture with damp hands and shape them into patties, set aside.

Place a large pan over medium heat, add coconut oil.

Fry patties in batches once oil is very hot for 8 minutes on each side.

# Calabacitas Quesadillas

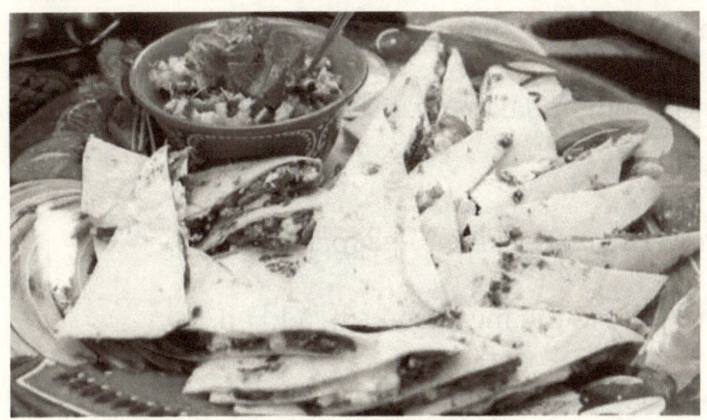

Cooking Time: 20 minutes

Servings: 2

Ingredients

2 large whole wheat tortillas

½ cup vegan Mexican shreds

½ onion, diced

1 jalapeno, seeded and diced

1 zucchini, quartered

kernels from 1 ear of sweet corn

1 teaspoon olive oil

2 cloves garlic, minced

¼ teaspoon cumin

salt and pepper

Instructions

Place a pan over medium heat. Add olive oil.

Add garlic, onion, jalapeno, zucchini, corn to the pan and cook for 6 minutes.

Season with cumin, salt and pepper. Set aside.

Return skillet to the medium heat, add oil.

Add wheat tortilla, onion-garlic mixture, top with vegetable shreds and cook tortilla for 3 minutes on each side until golden brown.

Remove from pan, cut into 4 pieces and serve with salsa and guacamole.

# Chickpea Avocado Salad Sandwich With Cranberries

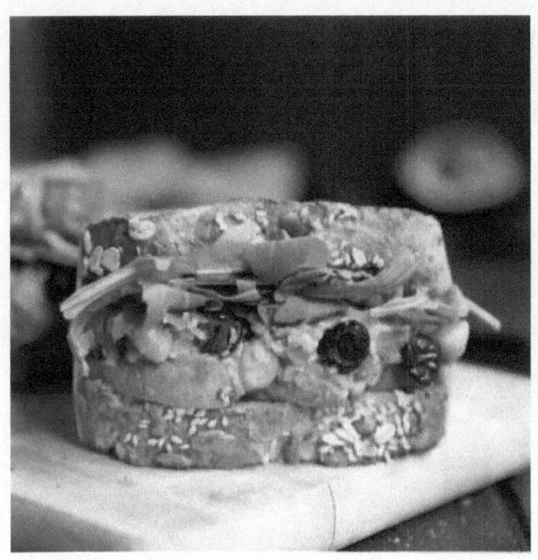

Cooking Time: 10 minutes

Servings: 2

Ingredients

15 oz. can chickpeas, rinsed and drained

¼ cup dried cranberries

1 large ripe avocado

4 slices gluten free bread, toasted

2 teaspoons freshly squeezed lemon juice

salt and pepper

Instructions

Combine chickpeas and avocado in a bowl, Mash until chunky in consistency.

Add lemon juice, cranberries, salt and pepper.

Spread the mixture on the toasted bread.

# Rice Paper Rolls with Mango and Mint

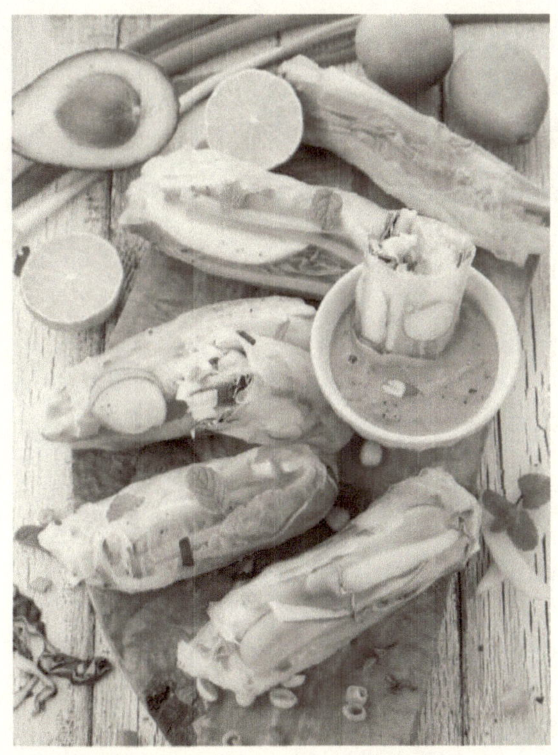

Cooking Time: 20 minutes

Servings: 6

Ingredients

For the rice paper rolls:

6 sheets Vietnamese rice paper

1 cup fresh mint

3 cups lettuce, thinly sliced

1 ½ cups glass noodles, cooked

1 cup purple cabbage, thinly sliced

1 avocado, thinly sliced

1 cucumber, chopped

3 carrots, thinly sliced

1 mango, thinly sliced

3 green onions, cut into rings

6 radishes, thinly sliced

For the fried sesame tofu:

7 oz. block firm tofu, thinly sliced

1 teaspoon sesame oil

1 tablespoon soy sauce

1 tablespoon sesame seeds

For the peanut dipping sauce:

¼ cup chunky peanut butter

2 teaspoons soy sauce

1 clove of garlic, minced

4 tablespoons warm water

½ teaspoons Sriracha sauce

Instructions

Add tap water to a large shallow bowl, dip rice papers, but not for too long.

Place a large skillet over medium heat, add sesame oil.

Add tofu, soy sauce to the pan and cook for about 5 minutes until browned.

Add sesame seeds and cook for 60 seconds.

Mix the peanut dipping sauce ingredients in a bowl and set aside.

Fill rice papers with vegetables and tofu. Wrap them like a burrito.

Serve rolls with a side of peanut dipping sauce.

# Turmeric Chickpea Salad Sandwich

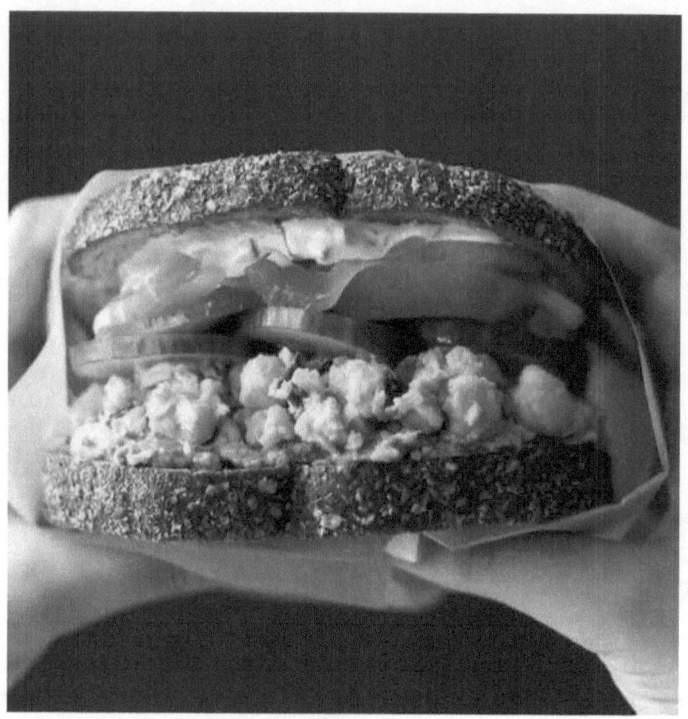

Cooking Time: 5 minutes

Servings: 1

Ingredients

1 can chickpeas, drained

1/3 cup aquafaba (liquid from the chickpea can)

½ teaspoon turmeric

½ teaspoon onion powder

1 clove garlic, minced

salt and black pepper

Instructions

Put all ingredients into a food processor and pulse until the consistency is chunky and not smooth.

Put in a bowl and serve.

# Mexican Quinoa

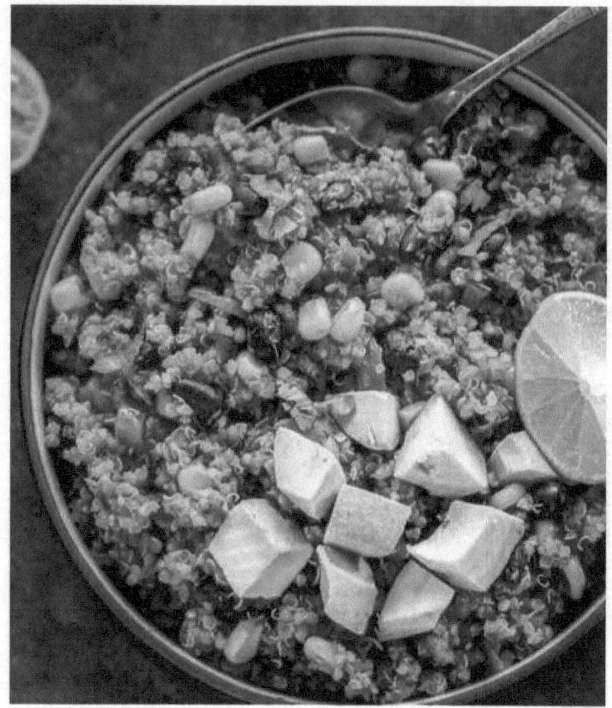

Cooking Time: 25 minutes

Servings: 4

Ingredients

1 cup quinoa, uncooked and rinsed

1 ½ cup vegetable broth

3 cups canned diced tomatoes

15 oz. can black beans, drained and rinsed

2 cups frozen corn

1 cup fresh parsley, chopped

1 onion, chopped

3 cloves of garlic, minced

2 bell peppers, chopped

1 tablespoon paprika powder

½ tablespoon cumin

2 tablespoons olive oil

2 tablespoons lime juice

2 green onions, chopped

salt and pepper

Instructions

Place a large pot over medium heat. Add olive oil.

Cook onions for 3 minutes.

Add garlic, bell peppers and cook for 5 minutes.

Add the remaining ingredients except lime juice, green onions and parsley. Cover and cook for about 20 minutes, keep checking to make sure the quinoa doesn't stick and burn.

Add lime juice, green onions and parsley.

Season the dish with salt and pepper before serving.

# Potato Fritters

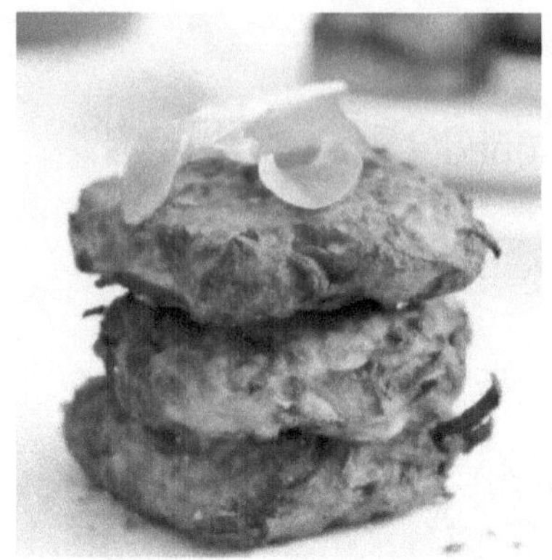

Cooking Time: 25 minutes

Servings: 12

Ingredients

For the vegetable potato fritters:

¾ cup red lentils, cooked

1 onion, chopped

2 cloves garlic, minced

2 potatoes, grated

1 carrot, grated

5 tablespoons all-purpose flour

½ teaspoon smoked paprika powder

1 teaspoon paprika powder

1 teaspoon majoram

salt and black pepper

For the Sriracha mayonnaise:

3 tablespoons vegan mayonnaise

1 teaspoon tomato paste

1 teaspoon garlic powder

½ teaspoon smoked paprika powder

Sriracha sauce

salt and pepper

Instructions

Add red lentils, carrot, potatoes, garlic, onion, flour, smoked paprika, regular paprika, Marjoram, salt and pepper to a large bowl.

Place a skillet over medium heat. Heat oil.

Scoop 2 tablespoons for each fritter and fry in the pan for about 4 minutes.

In a separate bowl combine Sriracha mayonnaise ingredients and set aside.

Serve fritters with salad and vegan sriracha mayonnaise.

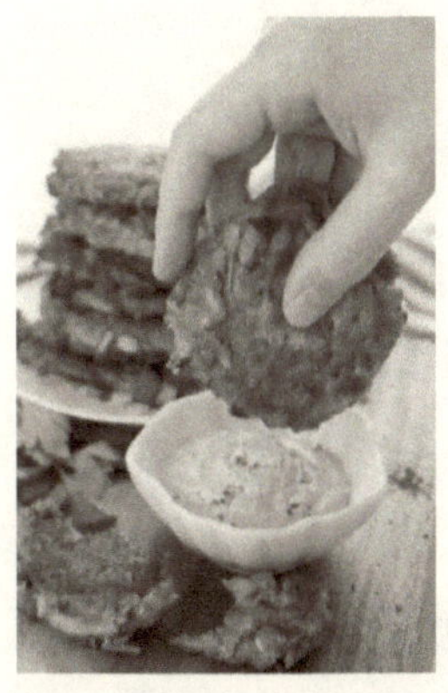

# Broccoli Pesto with Pasta and Cherry Tomatoes

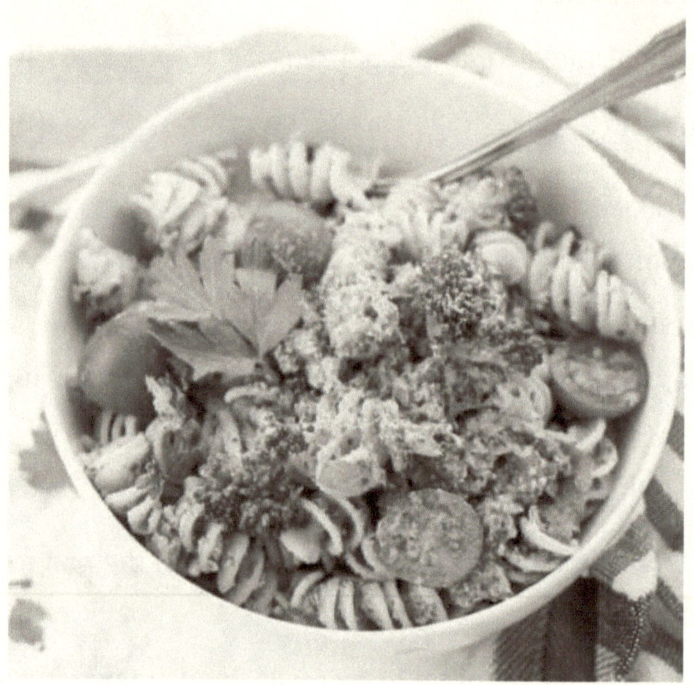

Cooking Time: 5 minutes

Servings: 2

Ingredients

For the broccoli pesto:

2 heaped cups broccoli florets, cooked

½ cup walnuts

3 tablespoons nutritional yeast

2 cloves of garlic

3 tablespoons olive oil

1/2 cup roughly chopped parsley

salt and black pepper

For the pasta:

9 oz. whole wheat pasta, cooked

1 cup cherry tomatoes, halved

1 cup cooked broccoli florets

Instructions

Combine pesto ingredients in a large bowl.

Serve cooked pasta with cherry tomatoes, cooked broccoli and pesto.

# Korean Barbecue Tempeh Wraps

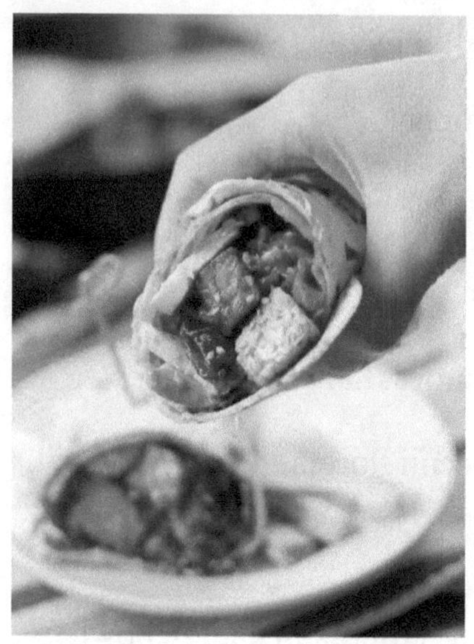

Cooking Time: 25 minutes

Servings: 4

Ingredients

For the Korean barbecue sauce:

¾ cup water

1/3 cup soy sauce

¼ cup maple syrup

¼ cup tomato paste

2 tablespoons gochujang

2 garlic cloves, minced

2 teaspoons ginger, grated

1 teaspoon sesame oil

For the Tempeh filling:

2 tablespoons vegetable oil

2-8 oz. packages tempeh, cubed

1 red bell pepper, thinly sliced

1 onion, thinly sliced

2 scallions, chopped

2 teaspoons sesame seeds

For the wraps:

4 large flour tortillas

4 large lettuce leaves

1 large avocado sliced

Instructions

Combine the Korean sauce ingredients in a bowl.

Place a large skillet over medium heat, add sauce and bring it to a simmer, lower the heat and let it simmer for 10 minutes.

Place another skillet over medium heat and add oil.

Add and cook tempeh for about 5 minutes.

Increase the heat, add bell pepper, onion and cook for 2 minutes, then lower the heat, add sauce and cook for 3 minutes. Once done, remove the from heat and set aside.

Put tortilla on a working surface, place lettuce leaves, avocado slices, and tempeh mixture on top. Wrap like a burrito to enclose the fillings inside

Do this for all tortillas before serving.

# Crab Cakes

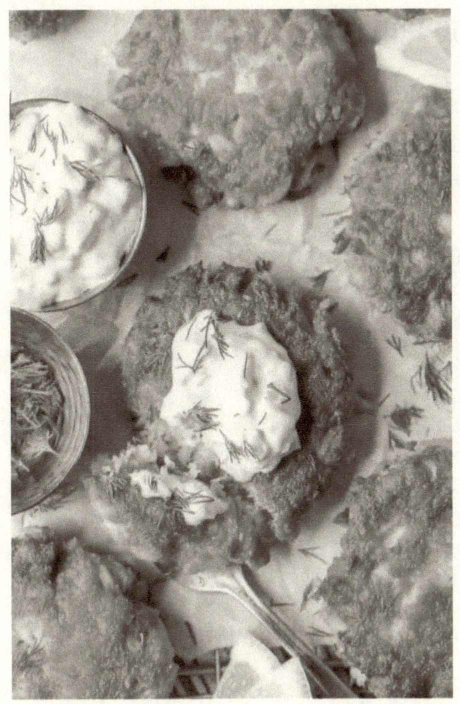

Cooking Time: 20 minutes

Servings: 8

Ingredients

2 cups cooked chickpeas

2 cans artichoke hearts in brine, drained and chopped

½ cup onion, chopped

¼ cup parsley, chopped

2 cloves garlic, minced

3 teaspoons fresh lemon juice

1 stalk celery, chopped

2 teaspoons Dijon mustard

3 tablespoons dill, chopped

1 cup panko bread crumbs

2 teaspoons vegan Worcestershire sauce

2 teaspoons fish seasoning

vegetable oil

salt and black pepper

Instructions

Place a skillet over medium heat. Add oil.

Sauté onions for about 2 minutes in the skillet.

Add garlic and cook 60 seconds. Remove from the heat and set aside.

Place cooked chickpeas in a bowl and mash them with a fork.

Add cooked onions, garlic and mix well.

Add the rest of the ingredients.

Season with salt and peppers. Form eight vegan crab cakes.

Place a skillet over medium heat add vegetable oil.

Add crab cakes and cook on each side for 3 minutes.

# **Smoky Black Beans Parsley Chimichurri**

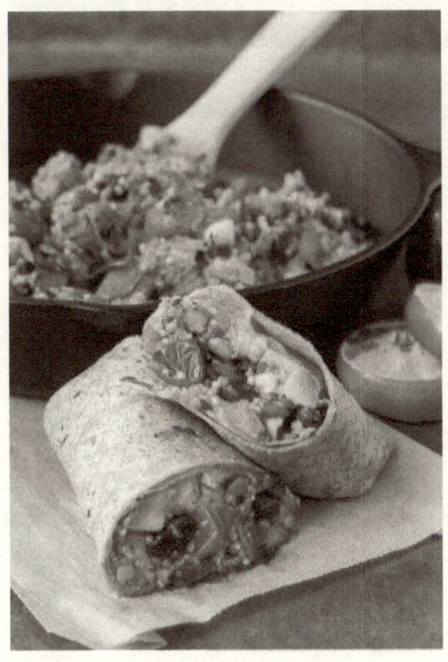

Cooking Time: 28 minutes

Servings: 3

Ingredients

For the smoky black beans:

2 teaspoons oil

15 oz. black beans

¼ cup onion, chopped

¼ cup bell pepper, chopped

2 cloves garlic, minced

½ teaspoon cumin powder

½ teaspoon chipotle chili pepper powder

½ teaspoon smoked paprika

1 medium tomato, chopped

½ zucchini, chopped

Other fillings:

Chimichurri

tortillas

2 cups baby spinach

2 red bell pepper, thinly sliced

Instructions

Place a large skillet over medium heat. Add oil.

Add and cook onions, garlic and bell peppers for about 8 minutes.

Add cumin, chili, smoked paprika, black beans, zucchini, tomato and salt. Mix, cover and cook on low medium for 10 minutes.

Place a large pan over medium heat and warm tortilla and spread Chimichurri on the tortilla.

Add black beans on the tortilla, cheese and sprinkle both bell peppers and spinach.

Wrap the tortilla before serving.

# Tuna Sandwich With Chickpeas

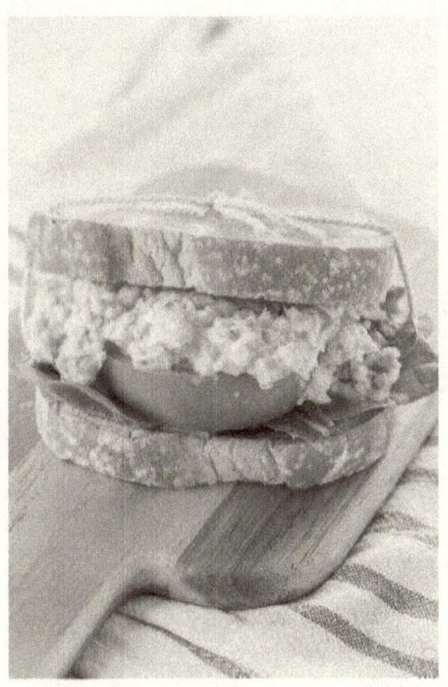

Cooking Time: 10 minutes

Servings: 2

Ingredients

For the vegan tuna salad:

1 can chickpeas

1 tablespoon dried Wakame seaweed

2 tablespoons vegan mayonnaise

1 teaspoon soy sauce

1 teaspoon lemon juice

2 teaspoons dill

2 stalks of celery, chopped

salt and pepper

For the sandwich:

4 slices of whole wheat bread

1 tomato, thinly sliced

¼ cucumber, thinly sliced

lettuce

½ onion, cut into rings

Instructions

Crumble the weed and place in a shallow bowl.

Add water and let the weed soak for 5 minutes. Drain excess water

Place chickpeas in a large bowl and mash it with a fork.

To the bowl, add celery, mayonnaise, dill, seaweed, lemon juice, soy sauce, salt and pepper and mix well.

## Sweet Potato Toast

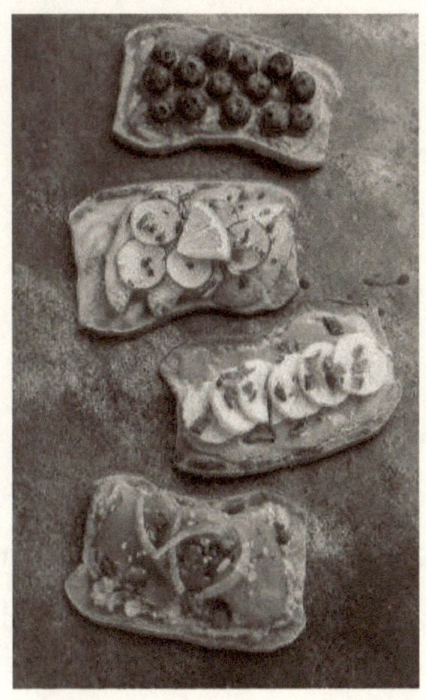

Cooking Time: 10 minutes

Servings: 1

Ingredients

1 medium sweet potato, washed and sliced to fit into the toaster

For the chickpea topping:

1 avocado

2 cups can chickpeas, drained and rinsed

½ teaspoon sumac

1 tablespoon lemon juice

½ cup small baby watercress

For the cashew cream pepper topping:

1/3 cup cashew cream

1 pepper, thinly sliced

1 handful baby basil leaves

cracked pepper to taste

olive oil to drizzle

Instructions

Place sweet potato slices in a toaster and toast on high. Then remove from the toaster and poke. Return slices to the toaster and toast again.

Combine avocado, sumac, chickpeas, salt and lemon juice in a bowl. Mash it all together.

When sweet potatoes are well toasted, transfer them to a plate.

Spoon the chickpea mixture and spread it on sweet potato slices.

Sprinkle baby watercress and smear cashew cream on top.

Follow with basil leaves, olive oil and cracked pepper.

# Cucumber Avocado Toast

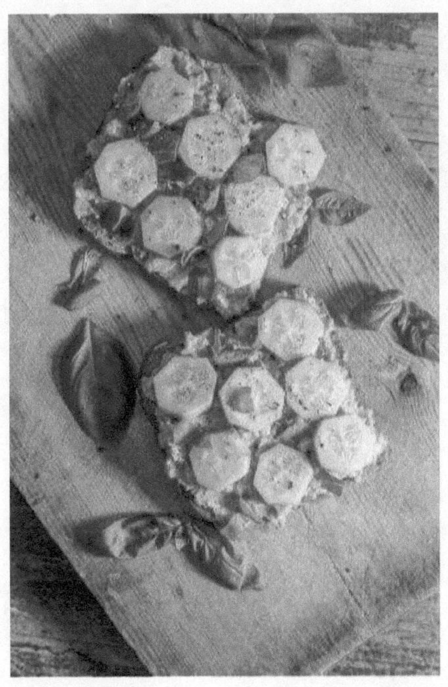

Cooking Time: 5 minutes

Servings: 2

Ingredients

1 cucumber, sliced

2 bread slices, toasted

¼ handful basil leaves, chopped

4 tablespoons avocado, mashed

Salt and pepper, to taste

1 teaspoon lemon juice

Instructions

1-Combine lemon juice together with the mashed avocado, and then spread the mixture on two bread slices.

2 -Top with cucumber slices along with the finely chopped basil leaves.

3-Generously sprinkle with salt and pepper and enjoy!

# Tofu Fish Sticks

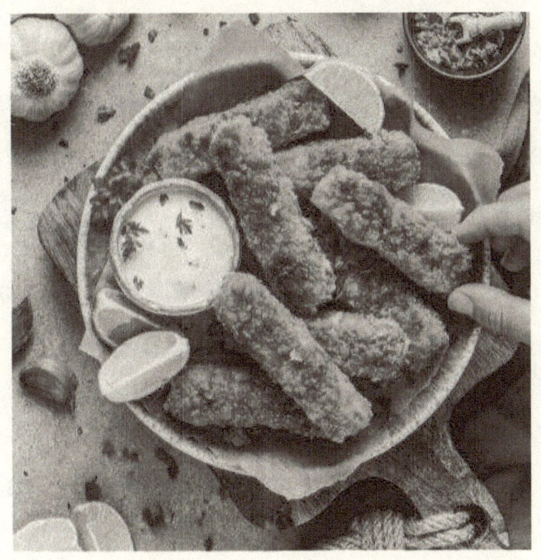

Cooking Time: 45 minutes

Servings: 4

Ingredients

1 cup bread crumbs

2 tablespoons nori seaweed, crumbled

2 blocks tofu, pressed

2 tablespoons soy sauce

1 teaspoon lemon pepper

1/4 cup soy milk

2 tablespoons lemon juice

Instructions

Preheat the oven to 375F and then cut the tofu into strips. Evenly coat the tofu strips with flour.

Whisk the soy milk together with soy sauce and lemon juice in a bowl, and then mix the lemon pepper, breadcrumbs and nori in a separate bowl.

When done, dip the tofu in the soy milk mixture and then coat the dipped tofu in the breadcrumb's mixture.

Bake for 40-45 minutes flipping only once, until crispy and brown. Alternatively, you can fry the both sides in the pan with little oil.

When baked through, serve and enjoy!

# Cornmeal Breaded Tofu

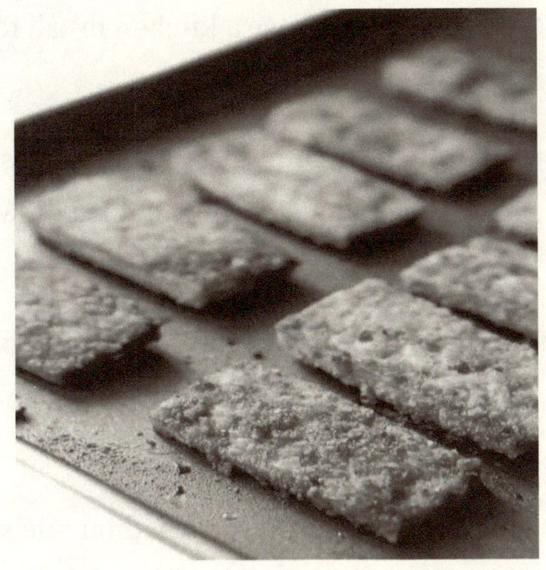

Cooking Time: 15 minutes

Servings: 4

Ingredients

1/4 cup cornmeal

1/4 teaspoon cayenne pepper

1 block tofu, pressed

1 teaspoon chili powder

2 tablespoons nutritional yeast

Salt and pepper, to taste

1/4 cup flour

Olive oil

Instructions

Preheat the oven to 400F and use a kitchen brush to lightly coat the baking sheet with oil.

Cut the pressed tofu into thin rectangular strips. Mix flour, nutritionist yeast, spices and cornmeal in a bowl until well combined.

Add the tofu pieces bit by bit into the cornmeal mixture to coat evenly, and then place the coated tofu pieces on a prepared baking sheet.

Bake for 5-7 minutes until lightly browned on one side. Flip the tofu and bake for 5 more minutes until baked through. Serve.

# Baked Sweet Potato Fries

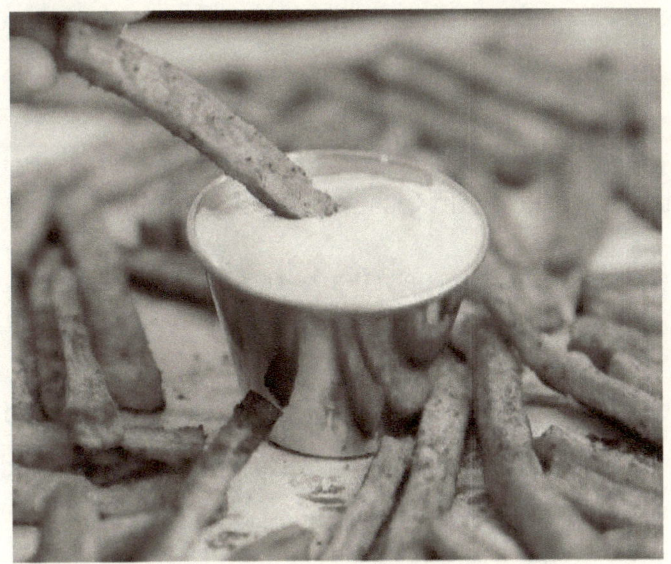

Cooking Time: 30 minutes

Servings: 6

Ingredients

1 tablespoon olive oil

3 large sweet potatoes, washed, peeled, chopped

1/4 teaspoon paprika

cooking spray

1 teaspoon cumin

½ teaspoon cayenne pepper

1/2 teaspoon salt

Instructions

Preheat the oven to 400F and prepare the sweet potatoes by washing and peeling them, and then chop the potatoes into wedges lengthwise.

Put the sweet potatoes wedges into a bowl and then generously drizzle them with oil and toss well until combined.

In a bowl, combine the paprika with salt and cumin, and then mix the ingredients together.

Sprinkle the cumin-paprika mixture on the sweet potato wedges and then toss well to combine, until the potatoes wedges are nicely coated with spices and olive oil.

Spray the baking sheet with cooking spray and then spread the coated sweet potatoes wedges in one layer on the sheet.

Bake the potatoes in the oven for 30 minutes.

When baked through, serve the sweet potatoes fries with your desired sauce and enjoy!

# Wheat Thins

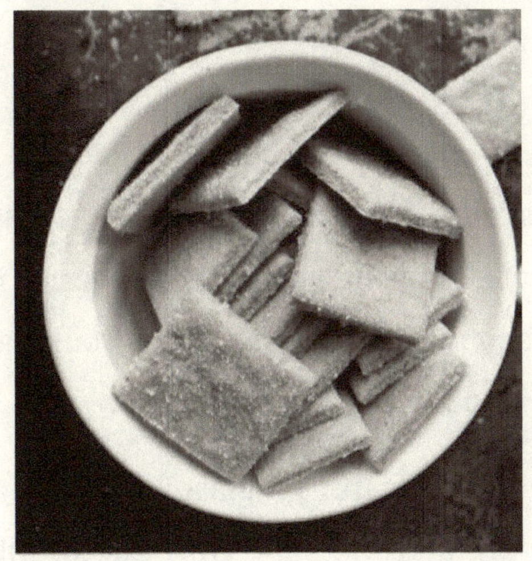

Cooking Time: 15 minutes

Servings: 8

Ingredients

3 oz. water

2 1/2 oz. sugar

1/2 teaspoon ground turmeric

1 oz. coconut oil

1/2 teaspoon tartar cream

5 oz. flour

¾ oz. wheat germ, toasted

1 1/2 oz. bread flour

1/4 teaspoon baking soda

1/4 oz. barley malt syrup

1/2 teaspoon salt

Instructions

Prepare the crackers. Preheat the oven to 350F and prepare two parchment sheets. Add the sugar, wheat germ, flour, turmeric, tartar cream, coconut oil, bread flour and baking soda to a food processor bowl and blend until combined.

Add the barley malt syrup to a glass bowl along with water to dissolve the syrup, and then add into the dry blended mixture and continue processing until stiff dough is formed.

Knead the dough lightly on the surface, and then separate the dough into two equal parts.

Put the cut parchment sheets on a working surface and sprinkle with flour, and then place one of the dough halves in the middle of the paper. Sprinkle the dough with flour and roll out into the rectangle.

Use a pizza cutter cut the dough into bite-size squares and then place the crackers on a sheet pan.

Sprinkle the crackers with salt and bake for about 12 minutes. Rotate the pan halfway.

Let the crackers cool to a room temperature. When done, serve and enjoy!

# Spinach and Artichoke Dip

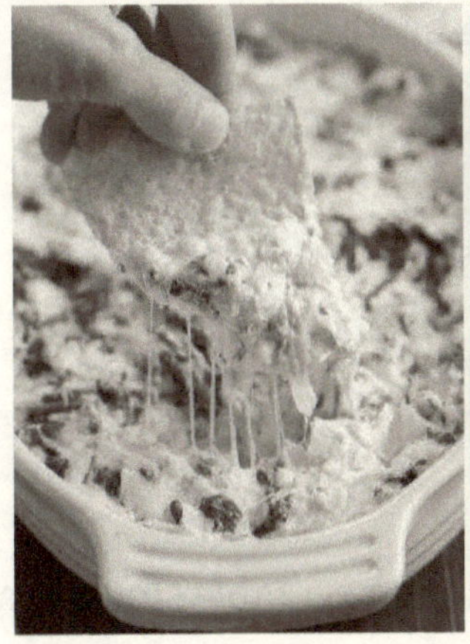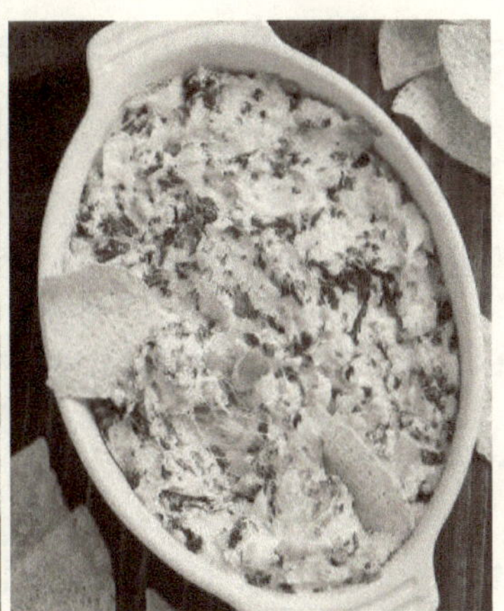

Cooking Time: 40 minutes

Servings: 6-8

Ingredients

2 tablespoons nutritional yeast

2 tablespoons olive oil

1 tablespoon Dijon mustard

1 lb. cauliflower, cored, chopped into florets

1 tablespoon lemon juice

1/4 cup vegan mayonnaise

10 oz. spinach

14 oz. artichokes drained, halved

2 oz. raw cashews

2 teaspoons garlic powder

1 cup vegetable stock or vegetable broth

2 garlic cloves, minced

Salt and pepper, to taste

Tortilla chips or pita chips, to serve

Instructions

Preheat the oven to 350F and add the vegetable stock to a skillet. Bring the vegetable stock to a simmer over medium heat and then add the cauliflower florets along with cashews and stir well until evenly coated. Set the heat to low and then close the lid. Cook for about 10 minutes until cauliflower florets are tender.

When done, transfer the cashews, cauliflower and the liquid to a blender and let cool for a minute. Process the mixture until smooth, and then add the nutritional yeast, mayonnaise, lemon juice, mustard and garlic powder, and continue processing until combined.

Use a kitchen towel to wipe the skillet and then add oil and heat on medium heat until warmed through. Add garlic and cook for 1-2 minutes until softened and fragrant, stirring frequently, and then add spinach along with salt. Continue cooking until the spinach wilts.

Add the cooked spinach to the blender along with the artichokes, and blend until incorporated.

Transfer the dip to a baking dish and bake for 30 minutes until the edges are slightly browned. Flip and bake the other side for about 2-3 minutes until nicely browned.

When baked through, serve immediately with chips and enjoy!

# Coconut Bacon

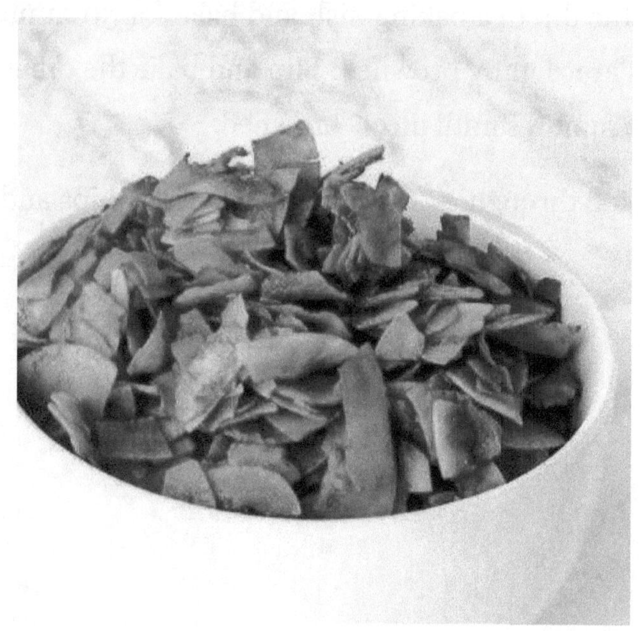

Cooking Time: 15 minutes

Servings: 6

Ingredients

1 teaspoon apple cider vinegar

2 tablespoons soy sauce or tamari

2 cups plain coconut flakes

2 tablespoons maple syrup

Pepper, to taste

1/2 teaspoon smoked paprika

Instructions

Preheat the oven to 325F and then add the coconut flakes to a mixing bowl.

Add all other ingredients to a separate bowl and then add the coconut flakes. Mix the ingredients together until the coconut flakes are evenly coated.

Spread the coated coconut flakes in one layer evenly on a baking sheet and bake for about 10 minutes. Stir and flip the coconut flakes, bake for 3-4 more minutes until nicely browned.

When baked through, remove from heat and let cool completely. Slice and serve.

# Baked Root Veg with Chili

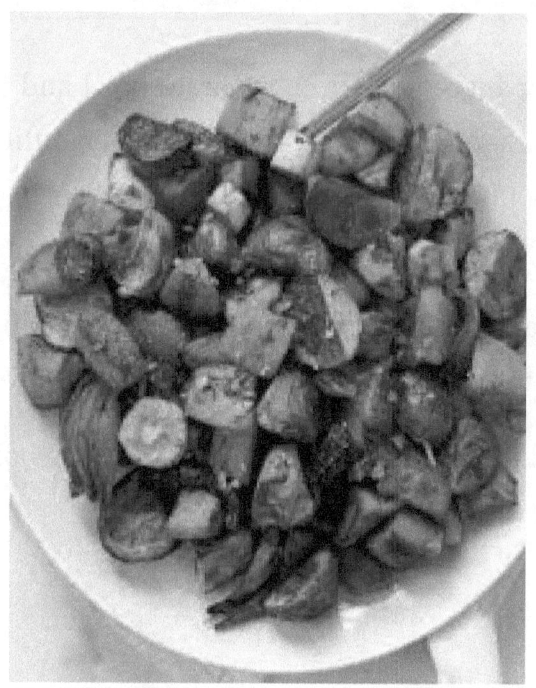

Preparation Time: 20 minutes

Servings: 2

Ingredients :

Potatoes (three medium)

Sweet potato (three medium)

Yam (three small)

Vegetable broth (two cups)

Red kidney beans (one can)

White kidney beans (one can)

Diced tomatoes (two cans)

Black beans (one can)

Dried oregano (one teaspoon)

Paprika (one and a half teaspoons)

Cumin (two teaspoons)

Chili powder (two tablespoons)

Celery (two stalks)

Carrots (two medium)

Bell pepper (one large red)

Red onion (two medium)

Olive oil (two tablespoons)

Cilantro (one bunch)

Avocado (two medium)

Bay leaf (one leaf)

Sweet corn (one can)

Tomato (two medium)

Lime juice (two medium)

Romaine (one head)

Directions:

Scrub and fork the potatoes and yams. Drizzle them with oil and quickly run over with clean hands. Sprinkle with salt and put on a baking tray for forty-five minutes or until you can pierce easily with a knife.

Heat the oil in a frying pan on medium and add the diced onion with the chopped bell pepper, diced carrots, and celery along with a quarter teaspoon of salt. Cook until the carrot is tender then add the paprika, oregano, cumin, and chili powder, along with the finely diced garlic.

Put in the full contents of the tomato cans, the bay leaf, and the vegetable broth.

Rinse all the cans of beans and drain well before adding to the pot. Stir the pot well and leave to simmer for a further thirty minutes. After this time has passed, get a potato masher and mash the chili to squish some of the beans and thicken the mixture.

At this point, you can add the juice of one lime, and salt and pepper to taste.

In separate bowls, prepare the fresh ingredients: finely dice the avocado and lightly mash with salt, pepper and the juice of another lime. Drain and rinse the corn and toss with half of the cilantro, finely chopped. Shred the romaine lettuce and dice the tomatoes.

Check that the root vegetables are done, remove from oven and slice open to cool slightly. Place in a nice dish and put on the table with a bowl of chili and all the sides for people to build their own masterpiece. You may also want to get vegan sour cream for this meal from the store. Enjoy!

# Autumn Stuffed Enchiladas

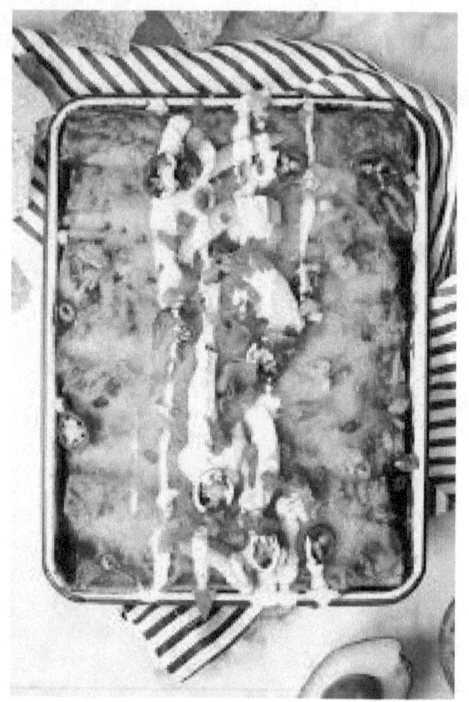

Preparation Time: 20 minutes

Servings: 2

Ingredients :

Salt and pepper (to taste)

Lemon juice (one medium lemon)

Cashews (one cup raw)

Cilantro (one bunch)

Roasted pumpkin seeds (quarter cup)

Corn tortillas (twelve pack)

Butternut squash (two cups)

Salsa (one and a half cups homemade or store-bought)

Black beans (one can)

Olive oil (two tablespoons)

Cayenne pepper (quarter teaspoon)

Chili flakes (one teaspoon)

Cumin (one teaspoon)

Garlic (three cloves)

Jalapeno (one medium)

Red onion (one small)

Brussel sprouts (one cup)

Direction :

Soak the cashews in boiled water to cover and set aside.

Cut the squash in half and after scooping out the seeds, lightly rub olive oil with clean hands over the exposed flesh. Sprinkle with a little salt and pepper before putting on a baking sheet face down. Cook for about forty-five minutes at 400F until it is cooked through.

Heat one tablespoon of olive oil in a frypan on medium heat and put chopped onion in, stirring until soft. Finely dice the jalapeno and garlic and finely slice the Brussel sprouts. Add these three things to the frypan and cook until the Brussels begin to wilt through.

Strain and rinse the black beans then add those to the frypan and mix well.

When the squash is cooked through and cool enough to handle, scrape out the soft insides away from the skin and put in a big bowl along with the Brussels mixture. Mix well again with the addition of generous pinches of salt and pepper to taste)

Put the tortillas in the oven to soften up (don't let them get crispy) while you get a baking dish out and very lightly oil the base and sides before spooning some salsa into it and doing the same. Spoon the squash mixture into the middle of the soft tortillas. Carefully roll them up to make little open-ended wraps, then put in the baking dish with the open ends down to stop them from unrolling.

Do this for all twelve tortillas then pour the rest of the salsa on top and spread to evenly coat. Change the temperature of the oven to 350F and bake for thirty minutes.

While these cooks put the drained, soaked cashews into a blender with one and a half cups cold water, lemon juice, and a quarter teaspoon salt. Blend until smooth, adding tiny drizzles of water if it becomes too thick. This is your sour cream.

When enchiladas are done, leave to cool while you chop cilantro. Then drizzle the sour cream generously over the dish and top with cilantro and pumpkin seeds. Enjoy!

# Creamy Vegetable Casserole

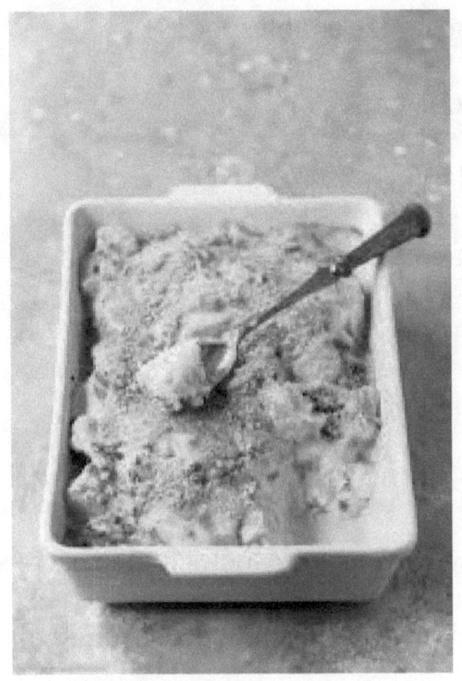

Preparation Time: 20 minutes

Servings: 2

Ingredients :

Fresh rosemary (two tablespoons)

Dried basil (one teaspoon)

Dried oregano (one teaspoon)

Garlic (three cloves)

Nutritional yeast (half cup)

Salt and pepper (to taste)

Olive oil (two tablespoons)

Apple cider vinegar (two tablespoons)

Raw cashews (one cup)

Zucchini (two large)

Broccoli (one medium head)

Cauliflower (one and a half medium head)

Russet potatoes (ten medium)

Directions:

Pour boiled water over the cashews and leave to soak.

Cut up the cauliflower into small florets and boil until soft.

The potatoes in this dish will be similar to scalloped potatoes so they need to be sliced thinly. Cut carefully, but don't be too precise, just so long as they are as thin as you can get them (think really fat potato chips).

When the cauliflower is done, drain it and put it in a blender along with the drained cashews and one and a half cups of cold water. Add a good half teaspoon of salt along with the apple cider vinegar and nutritional yeast. Blend until creamy.

Wash and grate the zucchini, set aside. Cut the broccoli into small bite-sized pieces and set aside.

In a large baking dish, spread the sides and bottom with generous amounts of olive oil. Then put two layers of potatoes down so that there are no gaps to the bottom.

Pour half of the cauliflower sauce to cover and spread evenly. Add the grated zucchini and spread out to cover the sauce. Sprinkle the oregano and basil over the zucchini, then push the pieces of broccoli into the zucchini to keep the surface as even as possible.

Drizzle a little more cauliflower sauce around the broccoli pieces to fill in the gaps. Do another layer to use up the rest of the potatoes, then pour the rest of the sauce over top of that. Spread it out as evenly as possible, right to the edges to fill in all the gaps around the sides.

Sprinkle the top with a half teaspoon of black pepper and a generous pinch or two of salt. Finely chop the fresh rosemary and sprinkle that on top also. Put in the oven on 400F for forty-five minutes. It will be done when a knife pierces the potatoes without pulling them up and the top should be beautifully browned. Let it cool before serving and enjoy!

Pasta – Italian, cheesy, decadent, lasagnas; all the words that mean love and care and satisfaction. These recipes will help you share the love with your guests and remind you what true self-love is when you make them for yourself. Indulgence doesn't have to be unhealthy.

# Butternut Squash Alfredo

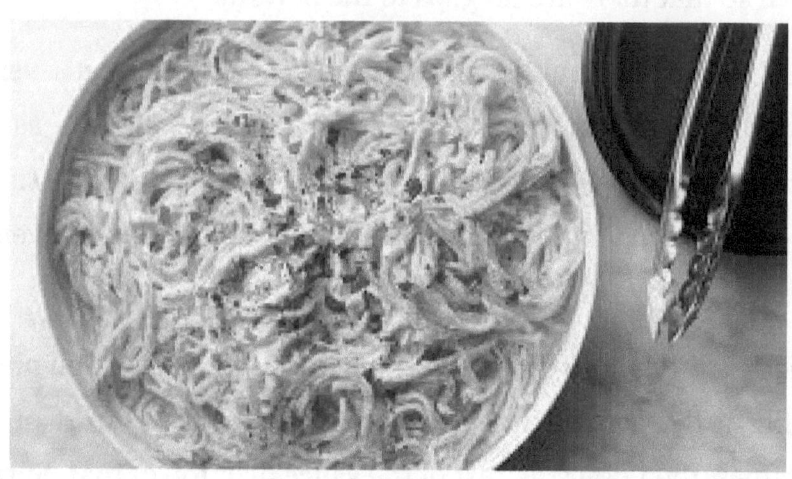

Ingredients :

Whole grain linguine (three cups)

Vegetable broth (two cups)

Butternut Squash (three cups diced)

Salt (quarter teaspoon)

Paprika (one teaspoon)

Black pepper (half teaspoon)

Garlic (two cloves)

White onion (one medium)

Green peas (one cup)

Zucchini (one large)

Olive oil (two tablespoons)

Sage (two tablespoons fresh)

Directions:

Heat the oil in a large frypan with medium heat. While it heats, ensures the sage leaves are clean and dry, then put in the oil to fry, moving around to not burn. Pull them out and put them on a paper towel.

Into the frypan, put the peeled and diced squash along with paprika, diced onion, and black pepper. Cook until the onion is soft then add the broth and salt to taste. Bring to a boil before turning down to low heat and leaving the squash to cook through.

In another pot, cook the linguine in water with a little salt.

When the squash is tender, put it in a blender along with all the liquid and other ingredients. Blend until creamy and taste to see if more salt, pepper or spice is needed. Put it back in the frypan to keep warm on low heat.

Using a grater, grate the zucchini lengthwise to make long noodles. Make as many long ones as you can to blend in with the linguine. Add them to the sauce along with the green peas and cook in the butternut squash for five minutes.

When the pasta is done, save one cup of liquid before you drain it. Add the linguine to the pasta and stir well to coat the linguine. If the sauce is too thick, add a little of the reserved pasta water.

Serve the pasta topped with the fried sage leaves and a little more black pepper. Enjoy!

# Vegan Lasagna

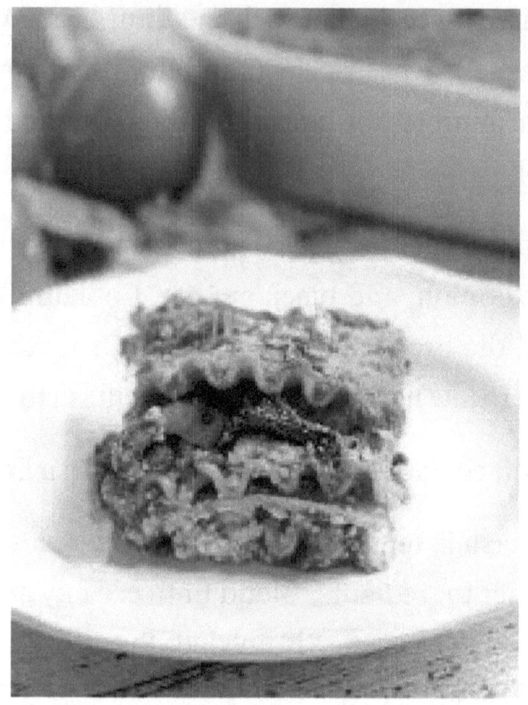

Preparation Time: 20 minutes

S erves: 2

Ingredients :

Tapioca starch (four tablespoons)

Salt (half teaspoon)

Apple cider vinegar (one tablespoon)

Lemon juice (four medium lemons)

Raw cashews (one and a half cups)

Baby spinach (three cups)

Lasagna noodles (one box)

Zucchini (two medium)

Garlic powder (half teaspoon)

Dried oregano (two teaspoons)

Dried basil (two teaspoons)

Salt (one teaspoon)

Olive oil (two tablespoons)

Nutritional yeast (half cup)

Firm tofu (one pack)

Tomato puree (one mini can)

Onion powder (one tablespoon)

Garlic (six bulbs)

White onion (one medium)

Salt and pepper (to taste)

Crushed tomatoes (two cans)

Dried red lentils (one cup dried)

Directions:

Put three cups of water in a saucepan with the lentils, then bring to a boil before reducing to a simmer for around twenty minutes. Drain the lentils and set aside.

In the same saucepan, add oil and the diced onion and let cook down. When the onion is soft, add finely diced garlic, generous pinches of salt and pepper, one teaspoon each of dried oregano and basil, the two cans of crushed tomato and the one can of tomato puree. Leave to simmer for fifteen minutes, stirring every five minutes. Add the lentils to this then set aside, this is the chunky marinara.

Put half a cup of cashews into a bowl with two cups of boiled water and set aside.

Wash and slice the zucchini into lengthwise strips that are long and relatively thin then set aside.

Put one cup of cashews in a blender and pulse until crumbly. Break up the tofu and add to the blender along with the juice from one lemon, one teaspoon each of basil and oregano, the nutritional yeast, garlic powder, and a little salt. Keep pulsing until it is mostly smooth but still a little textured. Put into a bowl and set aside, this is your ricotta.

Drain the soaked cashews and put them into a clean blender with the apple cider vinegar, the juice from one lemon, tapioca starch, and a little salt. Pour in one and a half cups of water and blend until smooth. Pour this into a saucepan on medium heat and stir until it becomes stretchy then set aside. This is the cheese sauce.

In a large baking dish, place a few spoonfuls of the marinara sauce and spread it to cover the bottom and sides of the dish. Begin to layer the lasagna noodles, the ricotta, the zucchini, and the cheese sauce. Follow this with half of the spinach, more marinara, lasagna noodles, ricotta, spinach, and the cheese sauce. Keep repeating until all ingredients have been used except for a small portion of the cheese sauce.

Put into a 350F oven for one hour on the highest shelf. Remove after forty minutes and spoon the remainder of the cheese sauce over the top to resemble mozzarella blobs, then return to the oven for twenty more minutes. Let rest then serve and enjoy!

# Creamy, Dreamy Dahl

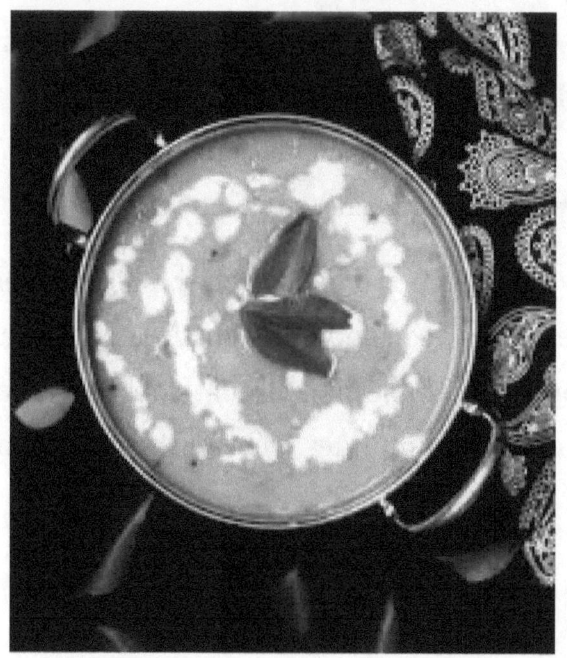

Preparation Time: 20 minutes

Servings: 2

Ingredients :

Fresh cilantro (small bunch)

Lemon juice (half one medium)

Red lentils (one cup dried)

Tomato (one medium)

Salt (three-quarter teaspoon)

Paprika (half teaspoon)

Ground cardamom (half teaspoon)

Turmeric (half teaspoon)

Fresh ginger (one tablespoon minced)

Garlic (four cloves)

Jalapeno (one medium)

White onion (two medium)

Cinnamon (one stick or quarter teaspoon ground)

Cumin (half teaspoon)

Coconut oil (two tablespoons)

Coconut milk (half can)

Basmati rice (one cup)

Directions:

Rinse the lentils then put in a saucepan with three cups of water and cook for twenty minutes on medium heat.

Chop the onion and finely dice the ginger, jalapeno, and garlic. Dice the tomatoes too and set aside.

Heat one tablespoon oil in a frypan on medium and put the cumin and cinnamon in the oil to release the aromas for one minute, then add the onions. Let them sweat a little before adding the garlic, ginger, and jalapeno.

In another saucepan, fill with rinsed rice, then top with water to cover. Add one tablespoon of coconut oil and the coconut milk (the liquid should be one inch above rice) and give it a quick stir. Cook on medium-high until it boils, then put the lid on and turn the heat down to medium-low and leave to simmer.

After a few minutes, put the salt, paprika, cardamom, and turmeric into the mix along with the diced tomato. If you used a cinnamon stick, pull it out now. Leave this on low to cook through.

When the lentils are done, drain them and put them back on the stove top. Scrape the tomato mixture into the lentils, along with the lemon juice and salt if needed. Mix well.

Check on the rice, and if the water has been absorbed and the rice can be easily fluffed up with a fork then it should be ready. Chop cilantro and top each serving of rice and dahl. Enjoy!

# Easy Thai Coconut Curry

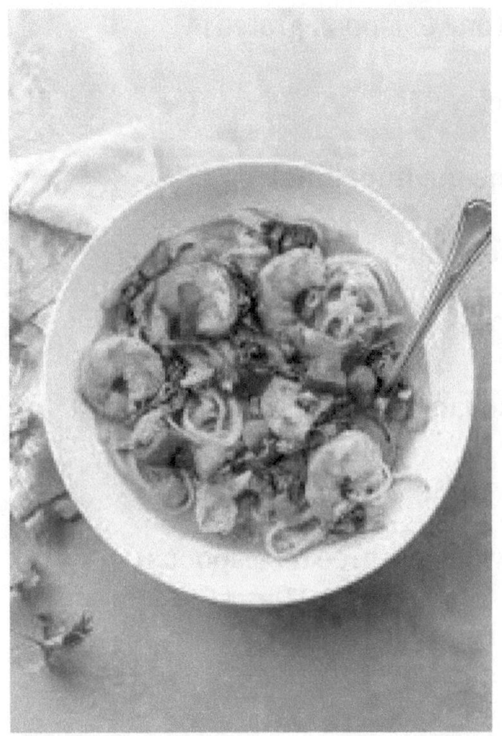

Preparation Time: 20 minutes

Servings: 2

Ingredients :

Jasmine rice (one cup)

Fresh basil leaves (quarter cup)

Kaffir lime leaves (three leaves)

Whole peppercorns (two tablespoons)

Snap peas (one cup)

Eggplant (one small)

Fresh ginger (one teaspoon grated)

Garlic (three cloves)

Lime juice (one medium lime)

Coconut oil (four tablespoons)

Maple syrup (one teaspoon)

Soy sauce (one tablespoon)

Firm tofu (one package)

Thai red curry paste (three tablespoons)

Coconut milk (one can)

Directions:

In a bowl, mix half the can of coconut milk with the soy sauce, maple syrup and curry paste.

Drain the tofu and cut into small cubes. Finely dice two cloves of garlic, grate the ginger and set aside. Cut the eggplant into small pieces, toss them in generous amounts of salt and set aside in a bowl.

In another saucepan, put one tablespoon coconut oil and heat on medium. Dice the last clove of garlic and put into the oil along with the rice. Stir around as the garlic cooks and the oil coats the rice. When some of the rice starts to get a little toasted, pour in water to just cover the rice and add the other half can of coconut milk along with one kefir lime leaf. Wait for it to come to a boil, then put the lid on, change heat to low and let it simmer without touching it.

Heat one tablespoon oil in a large frypan on medium and put in the tofu, cooking until all sides have been fried and are browned. Set the tofu aside.

Put in two more tablespoons of oil and put in the ginger and garlic and let fry for one minute. Rinse the salt off the eggplant, drain and put the eggplant in with the ginger and garlic.

When the eggplant gets a little soft and a little color, then add the snap peas and change heat to high. Put the curry mix into the pan and also the tofu and two of the lime leaves along with the peppercorns.

Cook for another two minutes while stirring to get everything coated and combined.

Check on the rice, it will be done when there is no liquid left and the rice can be fluffed easily with a fork. Remove the lime leaf and spoon rice onto plates.

Slice up the basil and quickly stir through the curry before spooning it over the rice. Finish with a generous squeeze of lime over everything and enjoy!

# Sabrosa Spanish Paella

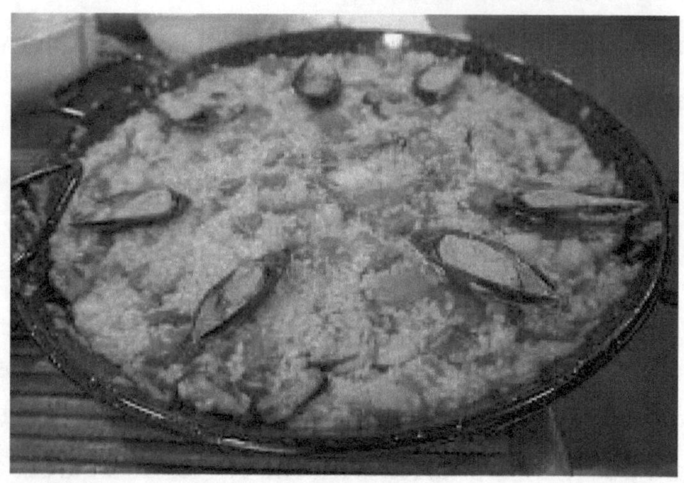

Preparation Time: 20 minutes

Servings: 2

Ingredients :

Paprika (one teaspoon)

Cayenne (half teaspoon)

Saffron (one pinch)

Capers (two tablespoons)

Garlic (two cloves)

Red bell pepper (three medium)

Artichoke hearts (two small jars)

Portobello mushrooms (three cups)

Lime (one medium)

White onion (one medium)

Salt and pepper (to taste)

Olive oil (three tablespoons)

Nutritional yeast (two tablespoons)

Saffron rice (two cups)

White wine (two cups)

Vegetable stock (six cups)

Directions:

Heat a large soup pot on medium-high and put in four cups of the vegetable stock and all of the wine. Let it boil before adding all the rice, then put the lid on and allow to simmer for fifteen minutes.

Turn on the oven at 375F.

Put two red bell peppers on a baking tray and cut them in half then rub with olive oil using clean hands so they are well coated. Put in the oven cut side down and cook for twenty minutes or until they get all wrinkly and start to look a little burnt.

Get an oven-safe large frypan (if you don't have one, then use a regular frypan and get an oven dish ready for later) and heat a tablespoon of olive oil on medium before adding diced onions and one thinly sliced bell pepper.

After the onions and bell pepper become soft, put in the sliced mushrooms and leave for five more minutes.

Put into the frypan the cayenne, paprika, and saffron and stir around. Then put in the finely diced garlic, capers and artichoke hearts (without the liquid).

When the bell peppers are ready from the oven, let them cool before pulling off their skins then chop them into small slices and add to the frypan.

Drain the rice and then put in the frypan and mix well. Add generous amounts of salt and pepper at this point and taste.

If you used an oven-safe frypan, then put it into the oven. If you didn't, then transfer the pan contents into an oven dish and put that in instead.

After ten minutes, pull out the dish and add one cup of vegetable broth and mix through really well. Do this again after another ten minutes, then remove ten minutes later. The paella should have been in the oven for a total of thirty minutes.

Cut up a lime into wedges and scatter about the dish. Roughly chop fresh parsley and scatter this over top also along with the nutritional yeast. Enjoy!

ROASTS – Going vegan doesn't mean you have to give up the traditional roast, if anything, it means you get to experience unique flavors and textures that you never knew existed!

# Vegan Festive Nut Roast

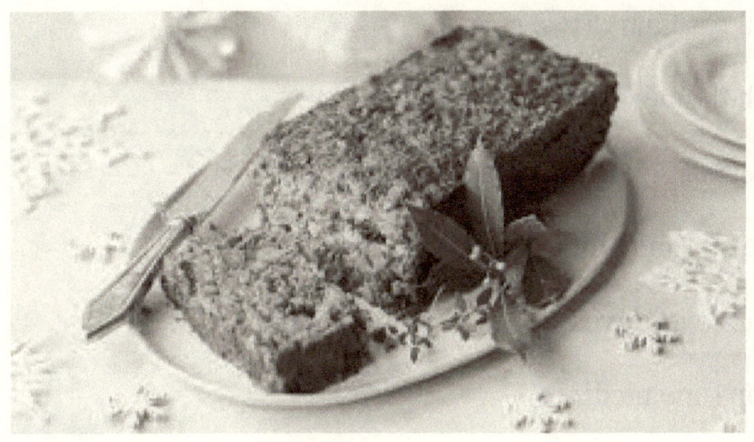

Preparation Time: 20 minutes

Servings: 2

Ingredients :

Paprika (two teaspoons)

Tomato puree (one teaspoon)

Miso paste (two teaspoons)

Dried rosemary (half teaspoon)

Dried sage (half teaspoon)

Dried thyme (half teaspoon)

Tahini (one tablespoon)

Dried breadcrumbs (one cup)

Chestnuts (one small can)

Raw cashews (one cup)

Carrots (one and a half cups)

Fresh rosemary (two sprigs)

Fresh thyme (two sprigs)

Butternut squash (one and a half cups)

Olive oil (one tablespoon)

Garlic (two cloves)

Onion (one medium)

Directions:

Peel and chop carrots and squash into small pieces then boil until they are very tender.

Put cashews and chestnuts into a blender and pulse until they are ground but not too fine.

Heat oil in a frypan over medium and put in chopped onion until softens. Finely dice garlic and put that in too.

Mash the carrots and squash in a bowl then add the onions and nuts. Mix very well then add every other ingredient. Well-oil a loaf sized dish and pack in firmly.

Bake at 350F covered with foil for one hour, then take off the foil and bake for another fifteen minutes.

Flip it out onto a plate and top with fresh thyme and rosemary, serve with cranberry sauce and mushroom gravy.

# Roasted Vegetable Pie

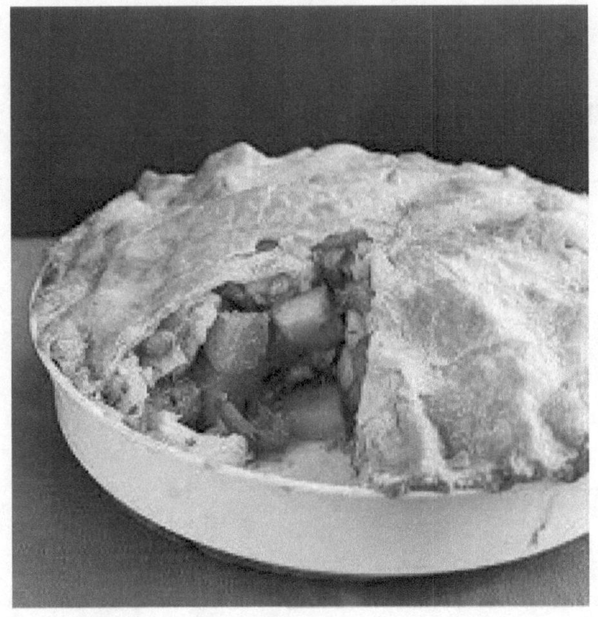

Preparation Time: 20 minutes

Servings: 2

Ingredients :

Vegetable suet or vegetable shortening (one cup)

White flour (one and two-thirds cup)

Salt and pepper (to taste)

Cranberry sauce (one tablespoon)

English mustard (one teaspoon)

Fresh thyme (two teaspoons)

Hazelnuts (one-third cup)

Chestnuts (one small can)

Butter beans (one can)

Dried cranberries (quarter cup)

Mushrooms (three cups)

Garlic (two cloves)

Olive oil (one tablespoon)

Leeks (one cup)

Onions (two medium)

Directions:

Heat oil in a frypan and put in the finely sliced leeks and onions. Let cook down for five minutes before adding the finely diced garlic. Put in the cranberries, drained and rinsed beans and chestnuts, chopped hazelnuts, sliced mushrooms, mustard, and thyme. Add generous pinches of salt and pepper then stir for ten minutes.

Sift flour and a half teaspoon of salt into a bowl and make a well in the middle.

Put two-thirds of a cup of water in a saucepan and bring to the boil then stir in the suet to melt.

Pour into the well of flour and gently fold the flour in until combined enough to knead. Do so for five minutes then set aside.

Oil a springform cake tin then roll out three-quarters of the pastry to lay into the tin. Spoon the cranberry sauce onto the base to cover then spoon in the vegetables.

Roll out the last quarter of the pastry and cover the vegetables. Run a knife around the edge of the lip to take off the extra pastry, then press down around the edges with a fork to pinch closed the top and base.

Drizzle and rub a tiny bit of oil over the top of the pie before you put it in the oven for one hour.

Let it sit for ten minutes before carefully lifting the sides of the cake tin and sliding the pie off the base onto a plate. Enjoy!

# Epic Vegan Holiday Roast

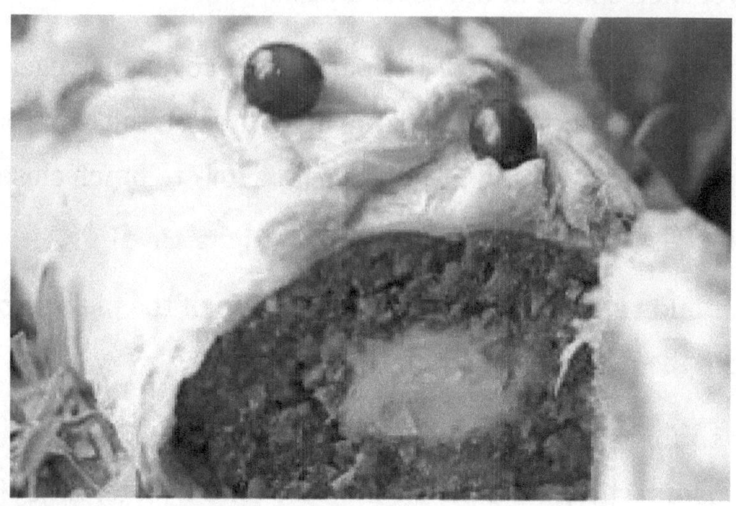

Preparation Time: 20 minutes

Servings: 2

Ingredients :

Salt and pepper (to taste)

Ground sage (three teaspoons)

Onion powder (three-quarter teaspoon)

Garlic powder (one teaspoon)

Soy sauce (one teaspoon)

Maple syrup (one teaspoon)

Miso paste (one tablespoon)

Olive oil (three tablespoons)

Pinto beans (half a can)

Vegetable broth (four cups)

Vital wheat gluten (two and quarter cups)

Sourdough bread (one small uncut round loaf)

Fresh parsley (half cup)

Fresh thyme (four sprigs)

Dried rosemary (one teaspoon)

Dried thyme (one tablespoon)

Mushrooms (four cups)

Garlic (five cloves)

Celery (one cup)

White onion (one large)

Barbeque sauce (two tablespoons)

Teriyaki sauce (two tablespoons)

Directions:

For the stuffing, dice the sourdough loaf into bite-sized chunks and spread over a baking tray. Bake for fifteen minutes at 350F tossing every five minutes.

Heat two tablespoons oil in a large frypan on medium and put diced onion and celery into it. When soft, add four cloves of diced garlic followed by diced mushrooms and another tablespoon of oil. Put in chopped fresh parsley with the dried rosemary, one tablespoon dried sage and the dried thyme.

When the mushrooms have cooked down, put in two cups of vegetable broth and generous sprinkles of salt and pepper. After it has simmered for five minutes, use a slotted spoon to pull out all the vegetables and put into a bowl with the bread chunks. Mix through really well then using a regular spoon, add the remaining liquid to the bread mixture until the bread has absorbed as much as it can without feeling soggy.

Oil a large baking dish and spread the contents into it before covering with aluminum wrap. Turn oven up to 375F and bake for thirty minutes covered and another twenty minutes uncovered. Set aside then turn the oven up again to 400F

In a blender put one teaspoon of sage with the onion and garlic powders. Put in one tablespoon of olive oil with the maple syrup, miso paste and one clove of whole garlic. Rinse the beans and put in along with one and a half cups of vegetable broth and one teaspoon of salt. Blend well until smooth and put into a big bowl then put in the vital wheat gluten and mix until it becomes dough-like. Use clean hands to work it (think of it like making bread) until it feels stretchy and uniforms then knead for another two minutes.

Use a rolling pin to roll it out to the size of your baking dish in a rectangle shape.

Spoon the stuffing down the center of the dough lengthwise. It should be stuffed so that when you roll it over, you have just enough dough left to pinch it together around the stuffing center. Do this the whole way down until you have a log. The stuffing should be densely packed inside so pack more in from each end if there's room.

Roll in oiled aluminum foil tightly and twist each end like a giant wrapped candy so that the roast is very tight. Put into a baking dish and pour the last half cup of broth around it like a bath and bake for ninety minutes but make sure you turn it every twenty minutes so that all sides get a chance on the bottom.

You know it's done when it feels firm to the touch much like a cooked meatloaf. Carefully unwrap the foil and put it back into the baking dish with a little drizzle of oil to stop it sticking.

Whisk together the BBQ and teriyaki sauces and pour over the roast making sure it is all coated. Put the fresh thyme sprigs on top and cook for a further ten minutes until the glaze gets sticky and darkens.

Let it rest for ten minutes then cut into rings and serve with mushroom gravy and cranberry sauce.

# Chapter 8: Dinner

## Butternut Squash Linguine With Fried Sage

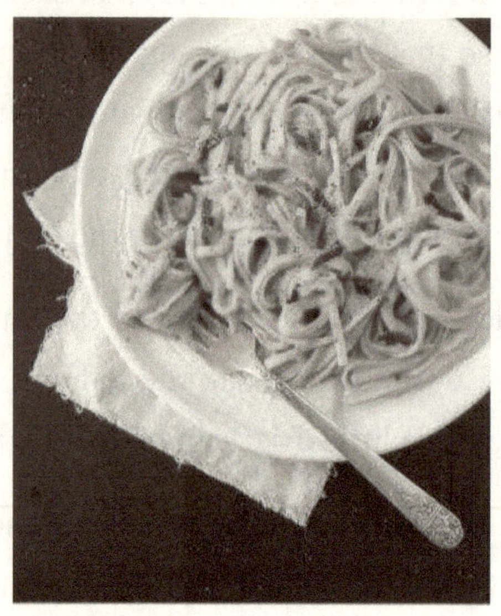

Cooking Time: 25 minutes

Servings: 4

Ingredients

3 cups butternut squash, peeled, seeded, and chopped

2 cups vegetable broth

12 oz. whole grain fettucine, cooked, 1 cup cooking liquid saved

1 onion, chopped

2 garlic cloves, pressed

2 tablespoons olive oil

1 tablespoon fresh sage, chopped

⅛ teaspoon red pepper flakes

salt and pepper

Instructions

Place a large pan over medium heat. Add oil.

Add sage and cook it until crispy. Season with salt and set aside.

Return the same pan to medium heat, add butternut, onion, garlic, red pepper flakes, salt and pepper. Cook for about 10 minutes.

Add broth and bring to a boil, then reduce the heat and let it cook for 20 minutes.

Place a pot of salty water over medium heat.

Cool the squash mixture and blend the mixture until smooth with a mixer.

Add pasta, ¼ cup reserved pasta liquid to the pan, return pan to medium heat and cook for 3 minutes.

# Paella

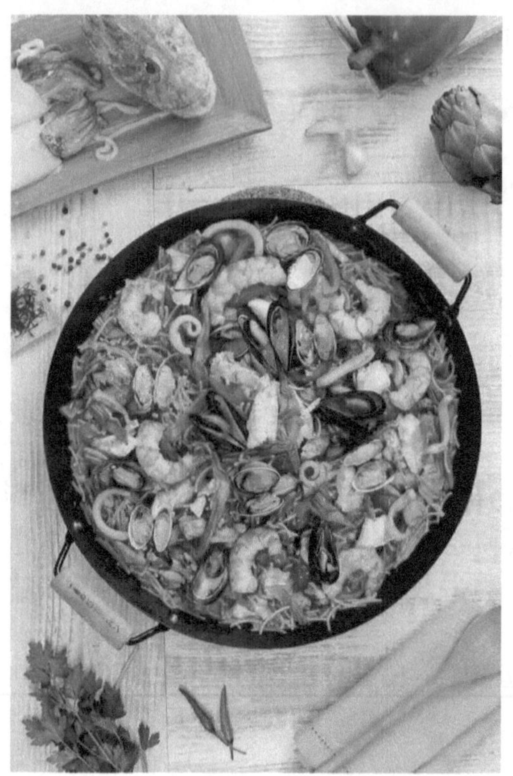

Cooking Time: 1 hour

Servings: 6

Ingredients

15 oz. diced tomatoes, drained

2 cups short-grain brown rice

1 ½ cups cooked chickpeas

3 cups vegetable broth

⅓ cup dry white wine

1 14 oz. artichokes, drained and chopped

½ cup Kalamata olives, pitted and halved

¼ cup parsley, chopped

½ cup peas

3 tablespoons extra-virgin olive oil, divided

1 onion, chopped

6 garlic cloves, pressed or minced

2 teaspoons smoked paprika

½ teaspoon saffron threads, crumbled

2 bell peppers, stemmed, seeded and sliced

2 tablespoons lemon juice

salt and pepper

Instructions

Preheat the oven to 350F.

Place a large skillet over medium heat and add 2 tablespoons oil.

Add onion, salt and cook for 5 minutes.

Add garlic, paprika and cook for ½ a minute.

Add tomatoes and stir well. Cook until the mixture starts to thicken.

Add rice and cook for 1 minute while stirring.

Add chickpeas, broth, wine, saffron and salt to taste. Increase the heat and bring the mixture to a boil. Remove from the heat.

Cover and immediately transfer to an oven on lower rack. Bake for 1 hour.

Prepare a baking sheet by lining it with parchment paper. Combine artichokes, peppers, olives, 1 tablespoon olive oil, salt and pepper. Mix well and roast vegetables on the upper rack in the oven for 45 minutes.

Add parsley and lemon juice to the baking pan and mix well.

Sprinkle the roasted vegetables and peas on the baked rice.

# Spicy Thai Peanut Sauce Over Roasted Sweet Potatoes and Rice

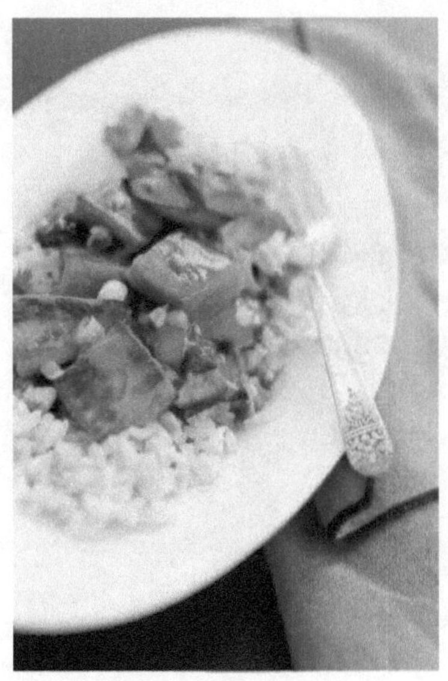

Cooking Time: 1 hour 30 minutes

Servings: 4

Ingredients

For the spicy Thai peanut sauce:

½ cup creamy peanut butter

¼ cup reduced-sodium tamari

3 tablespoons apple cider vinegar

2 tablespoons honey or maple syrup

1 teaspoon grated fresh ginger

2 cloves garlic, pressed

¼ teaspoon red pepper flakes

2 tablespoons water

For the roasted vegetables:

2 sweet potatoes, peeled and sliced

1 bell pepper, cored, deseeded, and sliced

about 2 tablespoons coconut oil (or olive oil)

¼ teaspoon cumin powder

salt

For the rice and garnishes:

1 ¼ cup jasmine brown rice

2 green onions, sliced

a handful of cilantro, torn

a handful of peanuts, crushed

Instructions

Place a pot of water on medium heat and bring it to a boil.

Preheat the oven to 425F.

On a rimmed baking sheet, mix sweet potato, 1 tablespoon coconut oil, cumin and salt. Roast in the middle rack for about 35 minutes.

On another baking sheet, mix bell pepper with 1 teaspoon coconut oil, salt and mix well, Roast on the top rack for about 20 minutes until tender.

When water is boiling in the pot add rice and mix well. Cook for about 30 minutes and drain excess liquid. Once done, cover and let it sit for 10 minutes, fluff it after.

Mix sauce ingredients in a small bowl and set aside.

Divide rice, roasted vegetables in bowls and top with sauce, green onions, cilantro and peanuts before serving.

# Butternut Squash Chipotle Chili With Avocado

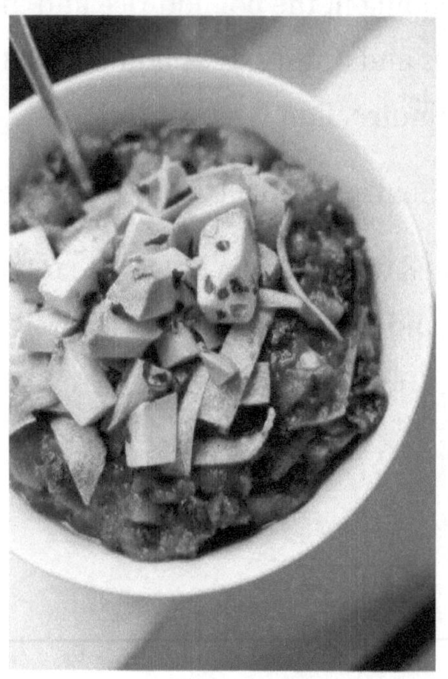

Cooking Time: 20 minutes

Servings: 4

Ingredients

3 cups black beans, cooked

14 oz. can diced tomatoes, including the liquid

2 cups vegetable broth

1 onion, chopped

2 bell peppers, chopped

1 small butternut squash, cubed

4 garlic cloves, minced

2 tablespoons olive oil

1 tablespoon chili powder

½ tablespoon chopped chipotle pepper in adobo

1 teaspoon ground cumin

¼ teaspoon ground cinnamon

1 bay leaf

2 avocados, diced

3 corn tortillas for crispy tortilla strips

salt

Instructions

Place a stockpot over medium heat. Add oil.

Add and cook onion, bell peppers and butternut squash for about 5 minutes.

Reduce the heat, add garlic, chili powder, ½ tablespoon chopped chipotle peppers, cumin and cinnamon. Cook for ½ a minute.

Add bay leaves, black beans, tomatoes and their juices and broth. Mix well. Cook for about 1 hour. Remove bay leaf when done cooking.

Slice corn tortillas into thin little strips.

Place a pan over medium heat and add olive oil. Add tortilla strips and season with salt. Cook until crispy for about 7 minutes. Remove from the heat and place in a bowl covered with paper towel to drain excess oil.

Serve chili in bowls, topped with crispy tortilla chips and avocado.

# Chickpea Biryani

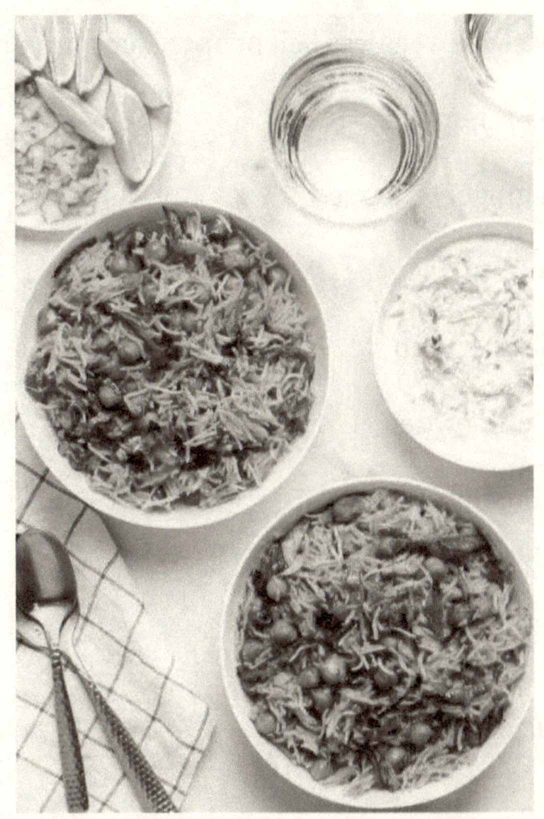

Cooking Time: 40 minutes

Servings: 6

Ingredients

4 cups veggie stock

2 cups basmati rice, rinsed

1 can chickpeas, drained, rinsed

½ cup raisins

1 large onion, thinly sliced

2 cups thinly sliced veggies (bell pepper, zucchini and carrots)

3 garlic cloves, chopped

1 tablespoon ginger, chopped

1 tablespoon cumin

1 tablespoon coriander

1 teaspoon chili powder

1 teaspoon cinnamon

½ teaspoon cardamom

½ teaspoon turmeric

2 tablespoons olive oil

1 bay leaf

salt

Instructions

Place a large skillet over medium high heat. Add oil.

Sauté onions for about 5 minutes.

Reduce the heat to medium, add vegetables, garlic and ginger. Cook for 5 minutes. Scoop 1 cup of this mixture and set aside.

Add spices, bay leaf and rice. Stir for about 1 minute.

Add stock and salt to taste.

Add chickpeas, raisins and 1 cup of vegetables. Bring the mixture to a simmer over high heat.

Lower the heat, cover tightly and let it simmer for ½ an hour. Remove from the heat when rice is done.

# Chinese Eggplant

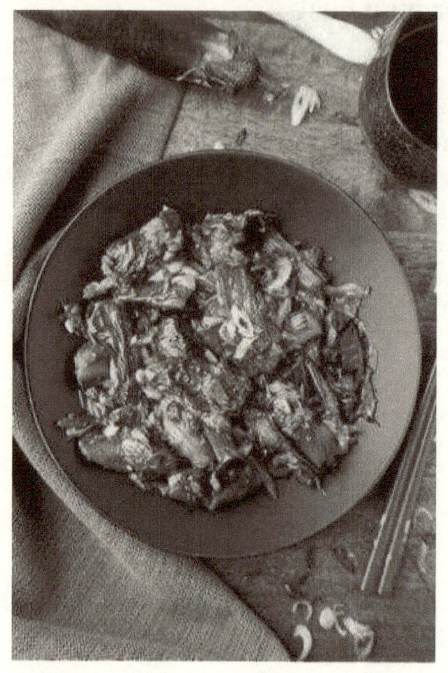

Cooking Time: 45 minutes

Servings: 4

Ingredients

1 ½ lbs. eggplants, chopped

2 cups water

2 tablespoons cornstarch

4 tablespoons peanut oil

4 cloves garlic, chopped

2 teaspoons ginger, minced

10 dried red chilies

salt

For the Szechuan sauce:

1 teaspoon Szechuan peppercorns

¼ cup soy sauce

1 tablespoon garlic chili paste

1 tablespoon sesame oil

1 tablespoon rice vinegar

1 tablespoon Chinese cooking wine

3 tablespoons coconut sugar

½ teaspoon five spice

Instructions

Place chopped eggplants in a shallow bowl. Add water and 2 teaspoons salt. Stir cover and let it sit for about 15 minutes.

Meanwhile place a small pan over medium heat. Toast the Szechuan peppercorns for about 2 minutes and crush them.

Add crushed peppercorns to a medium bowl, add soy, chili paste, sesame oil, rice vinegar, Chinese cooking vinegar, coconut sugar and five spice.

Drain excess liquid from the eggplants and toss in the corn starch.

Place a large skillet over medium heat, add eggplants and cook them until golden. Set aside.

Add 1 tablespoon of oil in the skillet placed over medium heat. Cook garlic and ginger for 2 minutes.

Add dried chilies and cook for 1 minute. Add the Szechuan sauce and bring the mixture to a simmer in 20 seconds.

Add back eggplants and cook for about 60 seconds.

# Black Pepper Tofu with Bok Choy

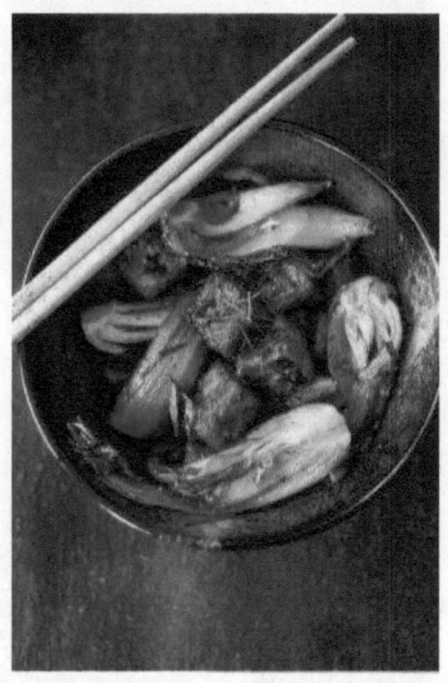

Cooking Time: 30 minutes

Servings: 2

Ingredients

12 oz. firm tofu, cubed

1/3 cup corn starch for dredging

2 tablespoons coconut oil

1 teaspoon fresh cracked peppercorns

1 shallot, sliced

4 cloves garlic, chopped

6 oz. baby bok choy, sliced to 4 slices

For the black pepper sauce:

2 tablespoons soy sauce

2 tablespoons Chinese cooking wine

2 tablespoons water

1 teaspoon brown sugar

½ teaspoon fresh cracked peppercorns

1 teaspoon chili paste

Instructions

In a small bowl, combine wok sauce ingredients and mix well until sugar dissolves. Set aside.

Place cornstarch in a shallow bowl and dredge tofu in the cornstarch. Set aside.

Place a large skillet over medium heat. Heat 1 tablespoon coconut oil.

Add peppercorns and toast for about 1 minute.

Add tofu and cook on all sides for about 6 minutes. Set tofu aside.

Add the remaining coconut oil. Add shallots, garlic and bok choy. Cook for 8 minutes.

Add back the tofu and cook for less than a minute.

# Spaghetti Alla Puttanesca

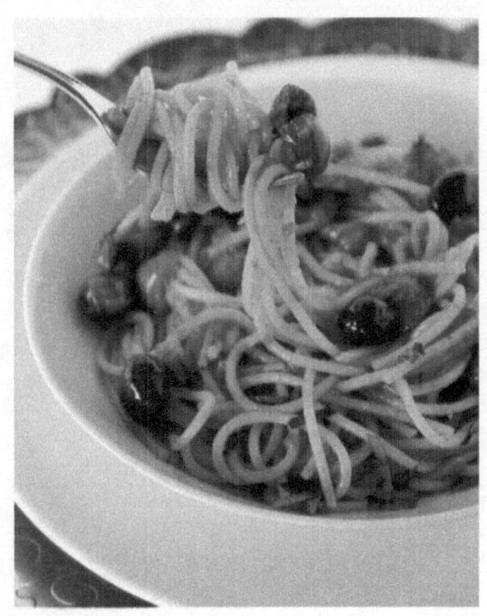

Cooking Time: 30 minutes

Servings: 4

Ingredients For the Puttanesca sauce:

28 oz. can chunky tomato sauce

⅓ cup chopped Kalamata olives

⅓ cup capers

1 tablespoon Kalamata olive brine

1 tablespoon caper brine

3 cloves garlic, minced

¼ teaspoon red pepper flakes

1 tablespoon olive oil

½ cup parsley leaves, chopped and divided

salt and pepper

For the pasta:

8 oz. whole grain spaghetti

6 oz. zucchini noodles

Instructions

Place a medium skillet over medium heat.

Add tomato sauce, olives, capers, olive brine, caper brine, garlic and red pepper flakes. Bring the mixture to a boil, reduce the heat and let it simmer for 20 minutes. Remove from the heat and set aside.

Place a pot over medium heat. Add water, salt, spaghetti and cook as directed on package. When done, drain excess water.

Pour the sauce over pasta and mix well.

Add zucchini noodles before serving.

# Thai Red Curry

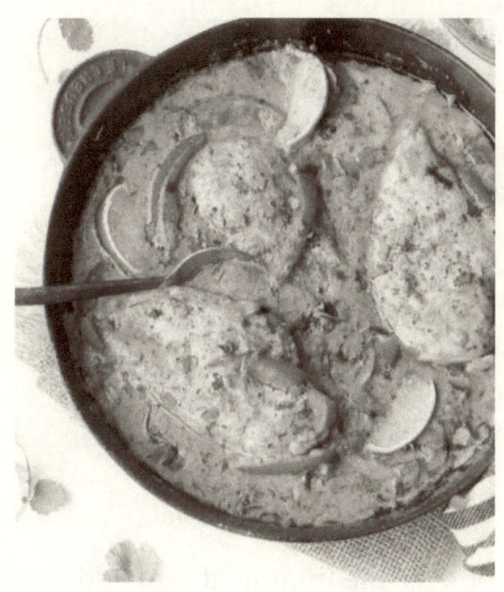

Cooking Time: 40 minutes

Servings: 4

Ingredients

1 ¼ cups brown jasmine rice, rinsed

1 tablespoon coconut oil

1 cup onion, chopped

1 tablespoon fresh ginger, ginger

2 cloves garlic, minced

1 red bell pepper, sliced

1 yellow bell pepper, sliced

3 carrots, peeled and sliced

2 tablespoons Thai red curry paste

1 14 oz. can coconut milk

½ cup water

1 ½ cups packed kale, chopped

1 ½ teaspoons coconut sugar

1 tablespoon tamari

2 teaspoons fresh lime juice

Instructions

Place a large pot over medium heat and add water. Bring it to a boil.

Add rice, salt and cook for 30 minutes. Remove from the heat, cover and let it sit for 10 minutes.

Place a large pan over medium heat. Add oil.

Cook onion and salt for about 5 minutes.

Add garlic, ginger and cook for about ½ a minute.

Add bell peppers, carrots and cook for about 5 minutes.

Add curry paste and cook for additional 2 minutes.

Add coconut milk, water, kale, sugar, tamari and lime juice. Remove from the heat.

# Thai Green Curry with Spring Vegetables

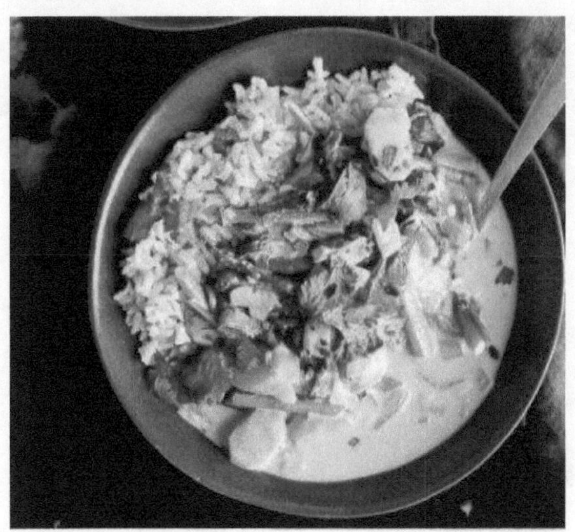

Cooking Time: 45 minutes

Servings:4

Ingredients

1 cup brown basmati rice, rinsed

2 teaspoons coconut oil

1 onion, diced

1 tablespoon fresh ginger, chopped

2 cloves garlic, chopped

2 cups asparagus, sliced

1 cup carrots, peeled and sliced

2 tablespoons Thai green curry paste

14 oz. full-fat coconut milk (I used full-fat coconut milk for a richer curry)

½ cup water

1 ½ teaspoons coconut sugar

2 cups packed baby spinach, chopped

1 ½ teaspoons fresh lime juice

1 ½ teaspoons tamari

salt

Instructions

Place a pot over medium heat. Add water and bring it to a boil.

Add rice, salt to taste and cook for 30 minutes. When done, cover the rice and set aside for more than 10 minutes.

Place a large skillet over medium heat. Add oil.

Cook onion, garlic, ginger and a pinch of salt.

Add asparagus, carrots and cook for 3 minutes.

Add curry paste and cook for additional 2 minutes.

Add coconut milk, ½ cup water, sugar and bring this mixture to a simmer. Reduce the heat and let it cook for 10 minutes until vegetables are tender.

Add spinach and let it cook for ½ a minute. Remove from the heat and season with rice vinegar and tamari.

# Tamarind Potato Curry

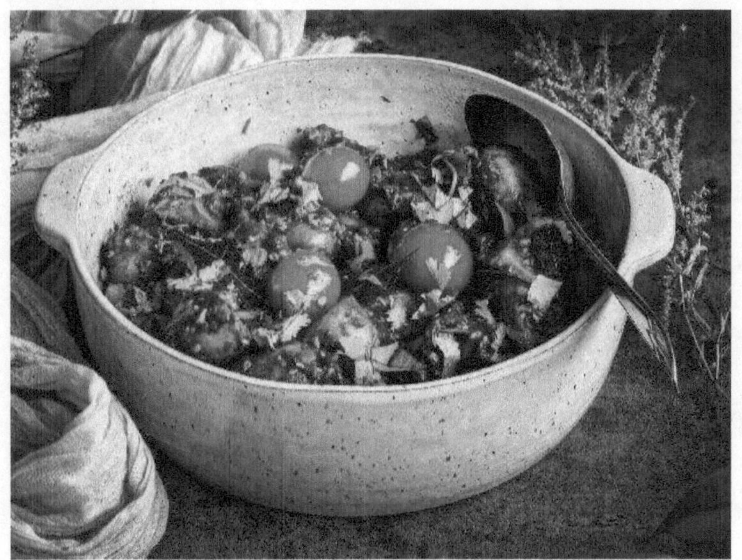

Cooking Time: 1 hour

Servings: 4

Ingredients

26.5 oz. potatoes, peeled and cubed

1 onion

1 garlic clove

1-inch ginger, chopped

1 green chilli, chopped

oil for frying

1 teaspoon cumin seeds

½ teaspoon fennel seeds

1 teaspoon ground coriander

1 teaspoon chilli powder

14 oz. plum tomatoes

2 teaspoon brown sugar

2 tablespoons tamarind paste

1 handful coriander leaves

rice or naan bread, to serve

Instructions

Place a pot of water over medium heat. Add salt and potatoes. Bring to a boil.

Place onion, garlic, ginger, chili, and 2 tablespoons water in a food processor. Pulse until smooth.

Place a pan over medium heat. Add oil.

Toast cumin and fennel seeds until they pop.

Add spices, puree and cook for 5 minutes.

Add tomatoes, sugar, tamarind and let it simmer for 10 minutes.

Add potatoes and some water. Cover and let it cook until tender.

Serve with rice or naan bread.

# West African Stew with Sweet Potato and Greens

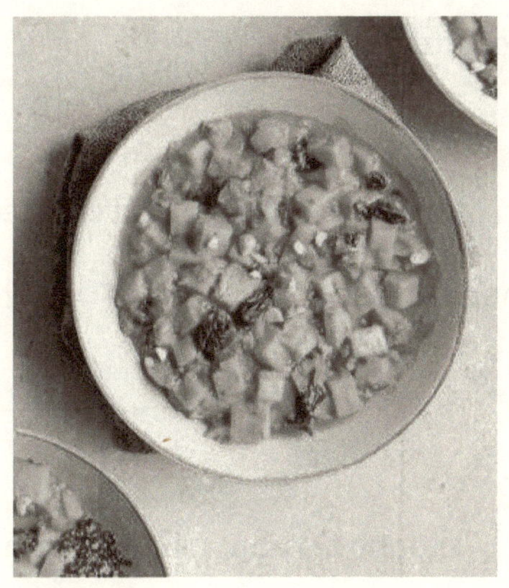

Cooking Time: 1 hour

Servings: 4

Ingredients

1/5 cup crunchy peanut butter

1/3 cup coconut cream

3 cups vegetable stock

21 oz. sweet potatoes, cubed

2 cups okra, halved

1 cup loosely packed kale, chopped

2 onions, 1 roughly chopped and 1 diced

1-inch ginger, chopped

3 garlic cloves

1 scotch bonnet chilli

4 tablespoons tomato purée

sunflower oil

2 teaspoons coriander seeds, toasted and crushed

2 teaspoons ground cumin

salt

Instructions

Combine roughly chopped onion, ginger, garlic, scotch bonnet, tomato puree and peanut butter in a blender. Blend for 1 minute until paste forms.

Place a cast iron pan over medium heat. Add 2 tablespoons sunflower oil.

Add diced onions and cook for 5 minutes. Season with salt.

Add spices, peanut sauce and cook for 5 minutes.

Add coconut cream, stock and bring it to a simmer for about 10 minutes.

Add cubed sweet potatoes, cover and cook for about 15 minutes.

Add okra, kale and cook for 10 additional minutes.

Remove from heat before serving.

## Kale Slaw

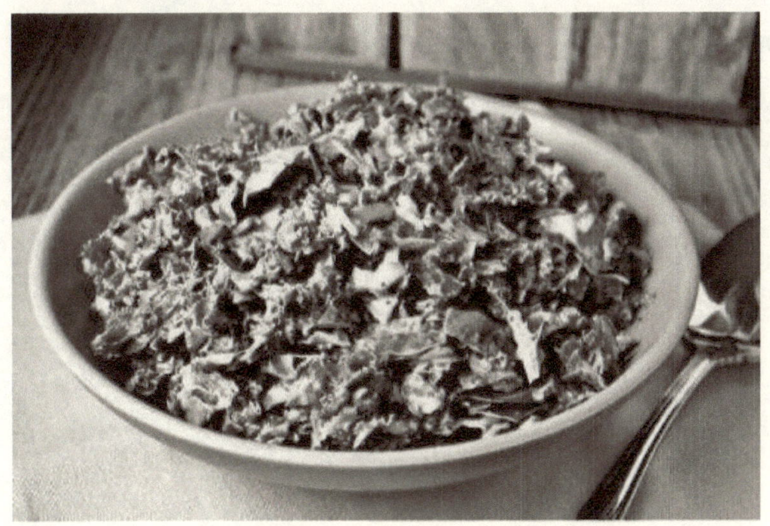

Cooking Time: 15 minutes

Servings: 4

Ingredients

1 small bunch kale, chopped

½ small head cabbage, shredded

¼ onion, thinly sliced

¼ cup tender herbs (cilantro, basil, parsley, chives)

¼ cup olive oil

4 tablespoons lemon juice

2 garlic cloves, minced

salt, pepper and chili flakes

Instructions

Combine kale, cabbage, herbs and onions in a large bowl.

Add olive oil, lemon juice, minced garlic, salt, pepper and mix
well.

Add chili flakes, toss well before serving.

# Moroccan Veggie Soup

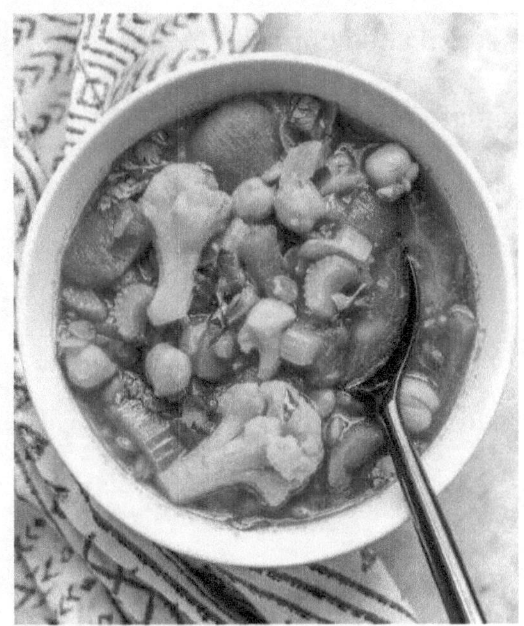

Cooking Time: 45 minutes

Servings: 4

Ingredients

1 2/3 cups chopped tomatoes

1 2/3 chickpeas, drained and rinsed

1 cup loosely spinach, chopped

2 teaspoons vegetable oil

1 onion, chopped

3 celery sticks, chopped

3 garlic cloves, chopped

2 preserved lemons, flesh discarded and rind finely chopped

2 red chili, deseeded and chopped

1 tablespoon tomato purée

2 teaspoons ground cumin

1 teaspoon ground turmeric

½ teaspoon ground cinnamon

1 potato, chopped

1 bunch flat-leaf parsley, chopped

4 tablespoons lemon juice

Instructions

Place a large pan over medium heat. Add onion celery and salt. Cover and cook for 10 minutes.

Add garlic, preserved lemons, red chilies and cook for 2 minutes.

Add tomato puree, spices and cook for 2 minutes.

Add chopped tomatoes, potato, chickpeas and 5 cups of boiling water. Bring to a boil and let it simmer for 30 minutes.

Add spinach, parsley and lemon juice before serving.

# Tex Mex Black Bean and Avocado Salad

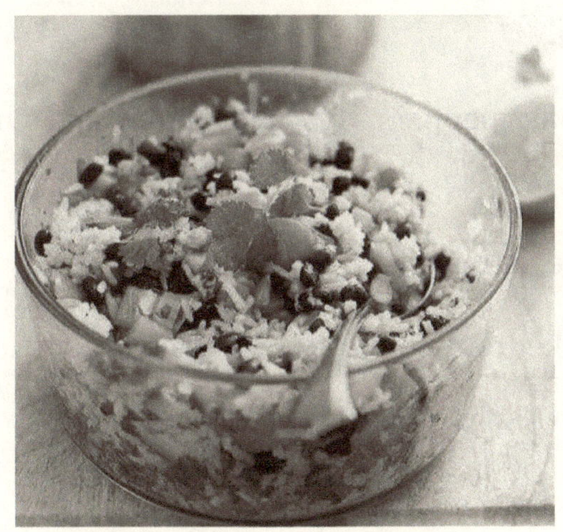

Cooking Time: 15 minutes

Servings: 2

Ingredients

14 oz. black beans, drained and rinsed

3 jars roasted red peppers, chopped

1 avocado, chopped

½ onion, chopped

1 red chili, chopped

1 lime, plus wedges to serve

olive oil

1 teaspoon cumin seeds

2 handfuls rocket

2 pitta breads, warmed

Instructions

Combine beans, peppers, avocado, onion and chili in a large mixing bowl.

Add lime juice, cumin seeds and mix well.

Serve the rocket on two plates with warm pittas and divide the bean mixture.

# Lentil Fattoush Salad

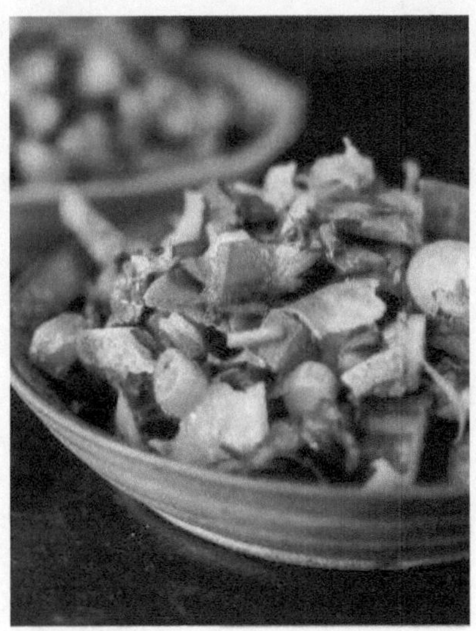

Cooking Time: 50 minutes

Servings: 2

Ingredients

⅓ cup dry green lentils

1 whole wheat pita pocket, chopped into bite sized pieces

2 teaspoons olive oil

2 teaspoons zaatar

4 cups loosely packed arugula

2 stalks celery, chopped

1 carrot stick, chopped

¼ small hothouse cucumber, chopped

1 small radish, thinly sliced

¼ cup dates, chopped

2 tablespoons toasted sunflower seeds

For the maple Dijon vinaigrette:

2 tablespoons olive oil

2 tablespoons balsamic vinegar

1 tablespoon Dijon mustard

1 tablespoon maple syrup

Instructions

Place a small pot over medium heat. Add lentils and 2/3 cup water.

Bring it to a boil, lower the heat and bring it to a simmer for 35 minutes. Remove from the heat and drain excess liquid.

Preheat the oven to 425F. Line a baking sheet with parchment paper.

Mix pita pieces with olive oil and zaatar. Place on a baking sheet and bake for 7 minutes.

Mix arugula, lentils, veggies, dates, sunflower seeds and pita croutons.

Meanwhile in a separate bowl, mix the dressing ingredients and set aside.

Add the dressing and toss well before serving.

# Sweet Potato Salad

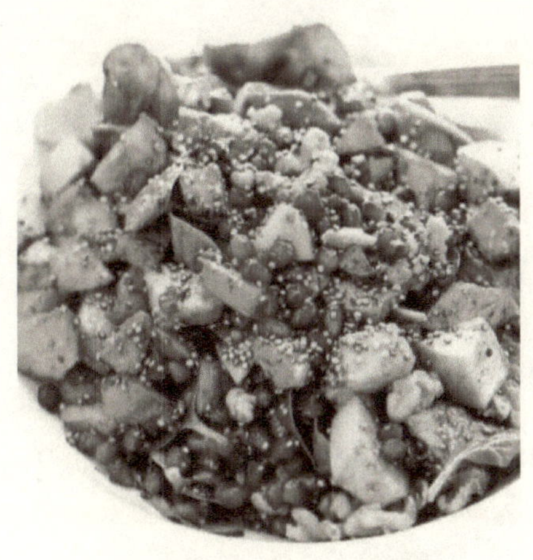

Cooking Time: 35 minutes

Servings: 4

Ingredients

2 sweet potatoes, peeled and cubed

1 tablespoon olive oil

½ teaspoon each of paprika, oregano and cayenne pepper

1 shallot, diced

2 spring onions, chopped

1 small bunch chives, chopped

3 tablespoons red wine vinegar

2 teaspoons olive oil

1 tablespoon pure maple syrup

salt and pepper

Instructions

Preheat the oven to 300F and prepare a baking sheet by lining it with parchment paper.

Place sweet potatoes in the baking sheet.

Drizzle some olive oil and spices, toss well and bake for 30 minutes.

In a separate bowl, mix shallots, scallions, chives, vinegar, olive oil and maple syrup.

Add baked sweet potatoes to the dressing.

# Lentil Salad with Spinach and Pomegranate

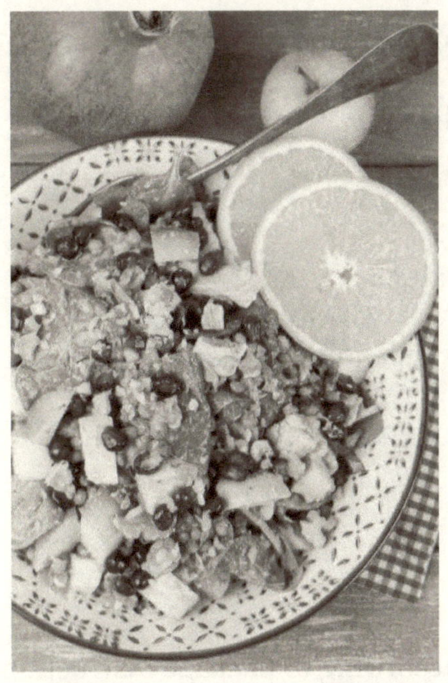

Cooking Time: 15 minutes

Servings: 3

Ingredients

For the vegan lentil salad:

3 cups brown lentils, cooked

1 avocado, cut into slices

2-3 handfuls fresh spinach

½ cup walnuts, chopped

2 apples, chopped

1 pomegranate

For the tahini orange dressing:

3 tablespoons tahini

2 tablespoons olive oil

1 clove of garlic

6 tablespoons water

4 tablespoons orange juice

2 teaspoons orange zest

salt and pepper

Instructions

Prepare lentils according to package instructions.

Place pomegranate in a shallow bowl filled with water, cut in half and take out seeds, remove fibers floating on the water.

Process all dressing ingredients in a food processor. Process until smooth and set aside.

Place salad ingredients in a large bowl and mix well.

Drizzle dressing over salad before serving.

# Broccoli Salad Curry Dressing

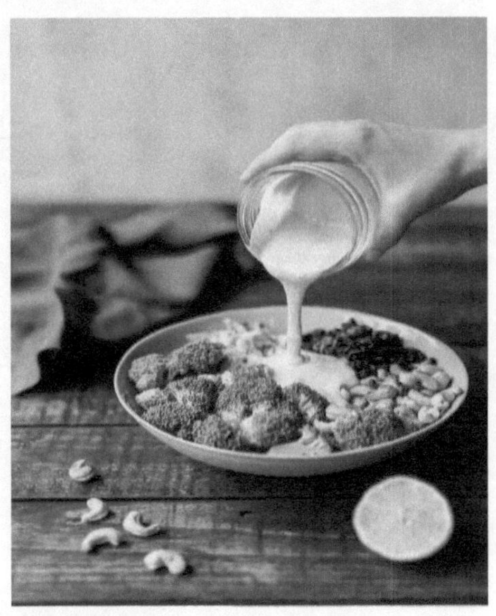

Cooking Time: 30 minutes

Servings: 6

Ingredients

½ cup plain, unsweetened vegan yogurt

¼ cup onion, chopped

2 heads broccoli florets, chopped

2 stalks celery, chopped

½ teaspoon curry powder

¼ teaspoon salt or to taste

2 tablespoons sunflower seeds

Instructions

Mix yoghurt, curry powder and salt.

Toss broccoli florets, celery onion and sunflower seeds.

Drizzle the dressing on top and put the salad in the fridge for 30 minutes.

# Broccoli Cauliflower Soup

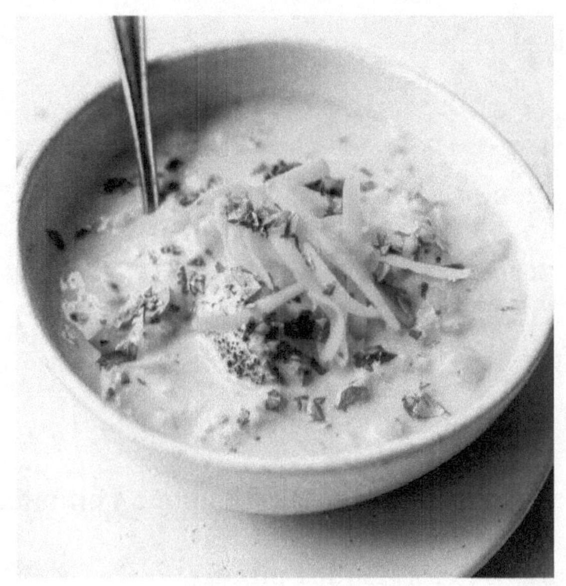

Cooking Time: 35 minutes

Servings: 8

Ingredients

1 medium head broccoli, finely chopped

1 medium head cauliflower, chopped

¼ cup whole wheat pastry flour

4 cups vegetable broth

1 cup unsweetened, unflavored almond milk

1/3 cup nutritional yeast

2 tablespoons olive oil

1 medium onion, chopped

2 cloves garlic, minced

2 carrots, diced

1 potato, diced

1 tablespoon lemon juice

salt and pepper

Instructions

Place a skillet over medium heat. Add oil.

Add and cook onion, salt, pepper for about 5 minutes.

Add garlic and cook for about 1 minute.

Add carrots, broccoli, cauliflower, potato and cook for 5 minutes.

Add flour and mix.

Add broth, almond milk, nutritional yeast and bring the mixture to a boil. Reduce the heat, cover and cook for 20 minutes. Remove from the heat and add lemon juice.

Use immersion blender to blend until chunky before serving.

# Carrot Ginger Soup

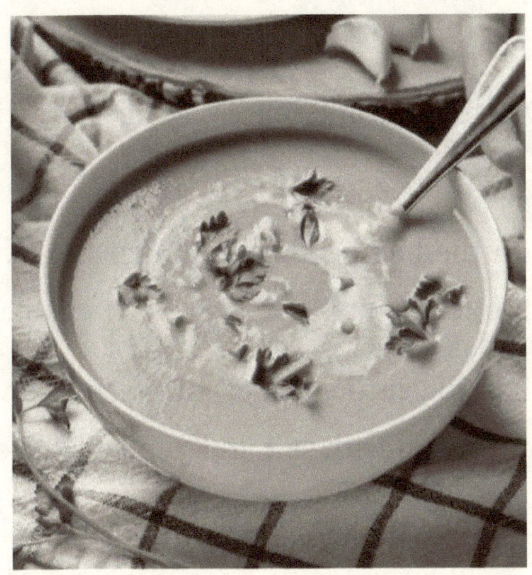

Cooking Time: 50 minutes

Servings: 6

Ingredients

1 lb. carrots, peeled and chopped

3 cups vegetable broth

1 cup vanilla almond milk

1 apple, diced

1 onion, diced

3 tablespoons avocado oil

1 teaspoon garlic, minced

1 tablespoon ginger, minced

½ teaspoon turmeric

Instructions

Preheat the oven to 425F and line a baking sheet with parchment paper.

Place carrots on the baking sheet and drizzle olive oil, salt and pepper. Bake for 30 minutes and set aside to cool.

Combine broth, milk, garlic, ginger, turmeric and vegetables in a food processor. Season with salt and pepper. Pulse until smooth and creamy.

Warm the creamy mixture with carrots on a stove before serving.

# Persimmon Butternut Squash Soup

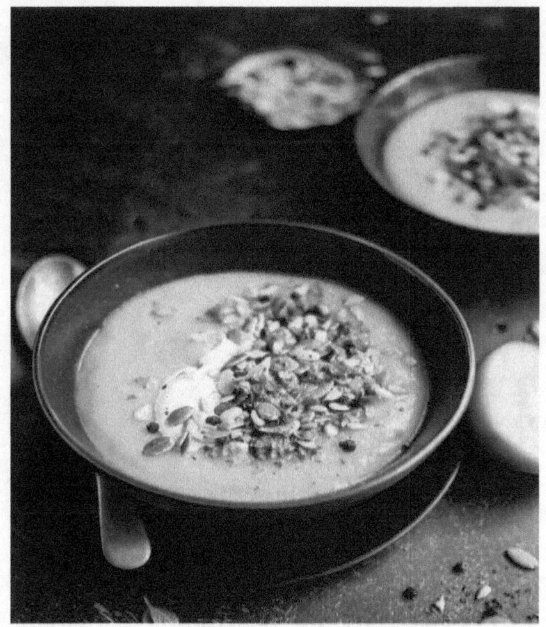

Cooking Time: 1 hour

Servings: 4

Ingredients

2 cups butternut squash, peeled and chopped

3 tablespoons olive oil

1 tablespoon butter

½ cup onion, chopped

3 persimmons, peeled and diced

18 oz. vegetable broth

1 cup coconut milk

1/8 teaspoon ground cloves

¼ teaspoon cinnamon

½ teaspoon paprika

¼ teaspoon ground ginger

1 tablespoon maple syrup

salt and pepper

Instructions

Preheat the oven to 400F, Line a baking sheet with parchment paper.

Place squash on the baking sheet and season with oil, cinnamon and salt. Bake for 25 minutes.

Meanwhile place a pot over medium heat.

Add butter and cook onions for 2 minutes.

Add squash, persimmon and cook for 5 minutes.

Add broth, milk, spices, maple syrup and bring it to a boil. Cover, reduce the heat and let it simmer for 20 minutes.

Remove from the heat and blend with an immersion blender until creamy and smooth.

Return to medium heat, add the remaining spices, salt and pepper before serving.

# Eggplant Tomato Soup

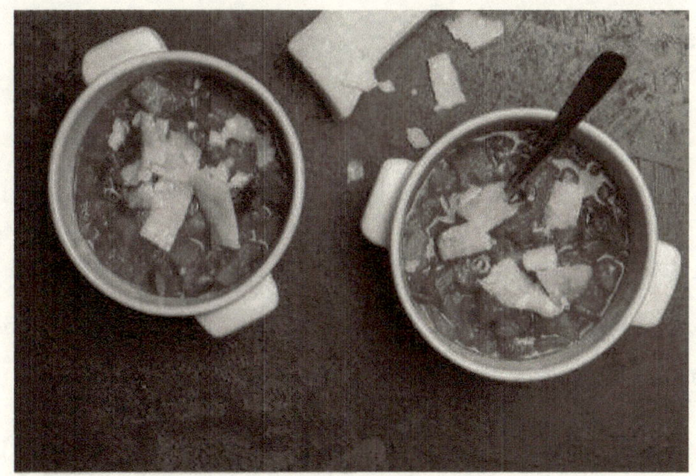

Cooking Time: 35 minutes

Servings: 4

Ingredients

½ cup raw cashews

1 eggplant, cubed

5 large tomatoes, cored and diced

1 onion, chopped

3 garlic cloves

¼ cup extra virgin olive oil

1 ½ cup vegetable broth

1 tablespoon tamari

1 tablespoon fresh oregano

1 tablespoon fresh basil

salt and pepper

Instructions

Preheat the oven to 400F and line a large baking sheet with foil.

Place a small pan over medium heat, add 2 cups water and bring it to a boil. Remove from the heat, add cashews and set aside to soak for 30 minutes.

Place eggplants, tomatoes, onion, garlic and a drizzle of olive oil, salt and pepper. Bake for 20 minutes until tender.

Place baked vegetables, soaked cashews, vegetable broth, tamari herbs and pulse for 1 minute until smooth.

Return to the skillet and heat the soup again before serving.

# Black Bean Soup

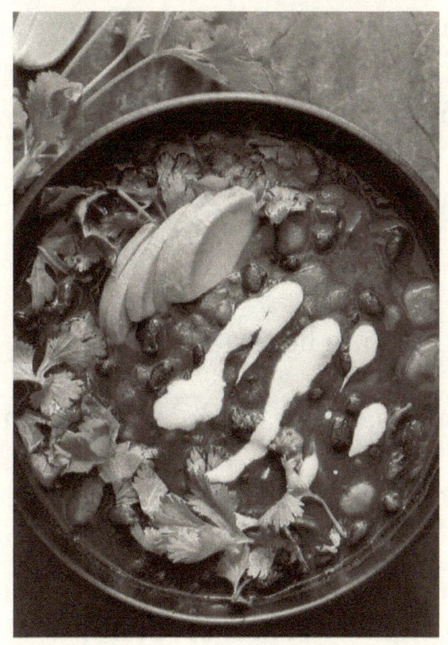

Cooking Time: 35 minutes

Servings: 4

Ingredients

3 15 oz. cans organic black beans

1 15 oz. can organic tomato sauce

¾ cup vegetable broth

1 teaspoon olive oil

1 white onion, chopped

3 cloves garlic, minced

1 ½ tablespoons chili powder

2 teaspoons cumin

1 teaspoon dried oregano

1/8 teaspoon cayenne pepper

salt

Instructions

Place a pot over medium heat, add oil.

Add and cook onions, garlic and cook for 5 minutes.

Add in chili powder, cumin, oregano, cayenne pepper and black pepper.

Add black beans, tomato sauce, broth and cook for 30 seconds. Bring to a boil, reduce the heat and let it simmer for 25 minutes.

# Veggieful' Chili

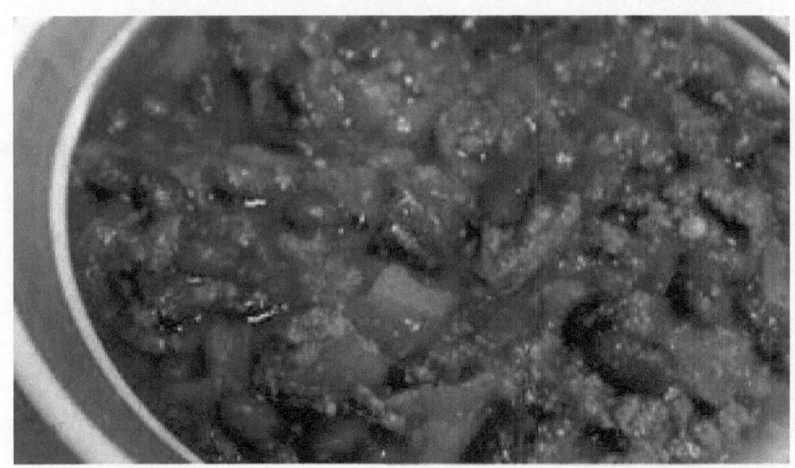

Servings: 8

Preparation Time: 15 minutes

Ingredients :

1½ cups raw black beans

1½ cups raw kidney beans

2 tbsp. olive oil

2 red onions (medium, diced)

1 clove garlic (minced)

2 tsp. cumin

¼ tsp. cayenne pepper

2 tsp. oregano

1 zucchini (medium, diced)

1 yellow squash (small, diced)

1 red bell pepper (small, diced)

2 cups water

1 jalapeño (medium, diced)

1 cup tomato paste

1 (200g) can sweet corn (drained)

1 tbsp. chili powder

Salt and pepper to taste

Directions:

Prepare the black and kidney beans according to the Directions.

Take a large pan, put it on medium high heat and add the olive oil.

Sautee the diced red onions for about 5 minutes.

Blend in the garlic, cumin, cayenne pepper, oregano while stirring.

Add the diced zucchini, squash, bell pepper and stir again.

Allow the mixture to fry for a few minutes while constantly stirring.

Lower the heat to medium and add 2 cups of water, jalapeño, tomato paste, corn and cooked beans.

Stir well while adding the chili powder, salt and optionally more pepper to taste.

Reduce the heat to low, cover the pan and let the chili simmer for about 20 minutes.

Add more spices like cumin, oregano, chili powder or cayenne pepper to taste.

Serve and enjoy warm or allow the chili to cool down to store it in containers!

# Red Curry Lentils

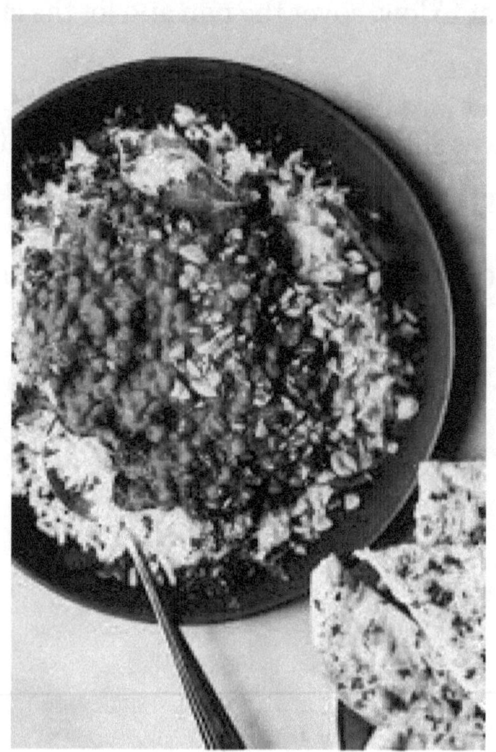

Servings: 6

Preparation Time: 20 minutes

Ingredients :

1 cup dry red lentils

2 tbsp. coconut oil

1 tbsp. cumin seeds

1 tbsp. coriander seeds

8 tomatoes (ripe, cubed)

1 head of garlic (chopped or minced)

2 tbsp. ginger (chopped)

1 tbsp. turmeric

1 tsp. cayenne powder

3 cups vegetable broth

2 tsp. sea salt

1 (15oz.) can coconut milk

½ cup cherry tomatoes

½ cup cilantro (chopped)

Directions:

Soak and drain the red lentils according to the Directions but do not cook them yet.

Put the coconut oil in a large pot heating over medium high heat.

Add the cumin and coriander seeds and garlic. Sauté the Ingredients for about 2 minutes while continuously stirring.

Add the freshly cut tomato cubes, ginger, turmeric and a pinch of salt to the pot.

Allow the mixture to gently cook, stirring occasionally for 5 minutes.

Blend in the red lentils, more salt to taste and cayenne powder.

Continue to add 3 cups of vegetable broth to the pot and allow the mixture to come to a soft boil.

Reduce the heat to low, cover the pot and allow the dish to simmer for about 30 minutes while stirring occasionally.

Once the lentils are soft, add the coconut milk and cherry tomatoes.

Bring the mixture back to a simmer before removing it from the heat and stir in the chopped cilantro.

Serve warm or allow the curry to cool down before storing.

Nutrition:

# Black-Bean Veggie Burritos

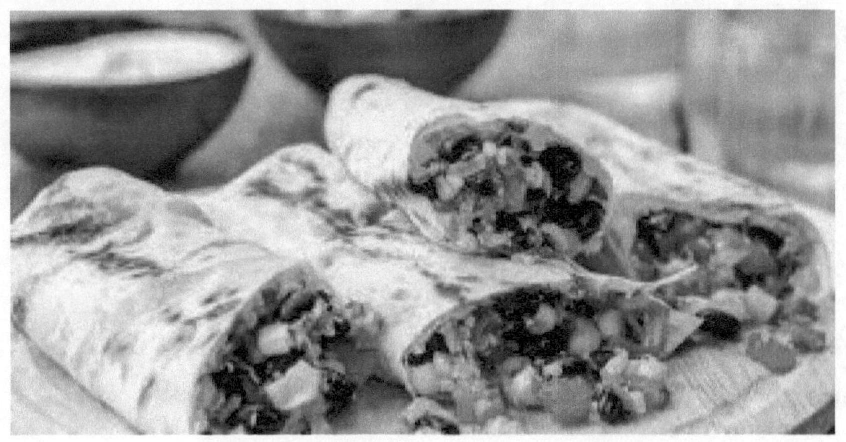

Servings: 8

Preparation Time: 30 minutes

Ingredients

For the filling:

2 cups dry black beans

1 tbsp. olive oil

1 red onion (diced)

1 zucchini (cubed)

1 red bell pepper (pitted, diced)

2 (150g) cans sweet corn (drained, rinsed)

¼ cup cilantro (chopped)

½ a lime (juiced)

Salt to taste

For homemade taco seasoning (optional)

1 tbsp. chili powder

2 tsp. ground cumin

½ tsp. paprika powder

¼ tsp. of each: garlic powder, onion powder, red pepper flakes, oregano, salt and cayenne

For the wraps:

8 tortilla wraps

½ cup no-salt vegan cream cheese

½ cup salsa

1 cup dry brown rice

Directions:

Cook the black beans according to the Directions.

Prepare the brown rice according to the recipe.

Mix all taco seasoning Ingredients in a bowl and set it aside.

Take a large pan, add the olive oil and put it on medium heat.

Add the diced red onion. Sauté for 3 minutes while stirring.

Add the zucchini and bell pepper and sauté for another 3 minutes.

Add in the black beans, corn and the homemade taco seasoning. Stir well and allow the mixture to simmer for about 10 minutes.

Turn off the heat and add the cilantro, lime juice and salt to taste.

Prepare the burrito by laying out a tortilla wrap and add the filling, salsa, rice and the optional vegan cheese.

Tightly wrap the burrito and place it back in the pan. Heat and press each side for about 2 minutes.

Serve warm or store each tortilla wrapped in aluminum foil in a Ziploc bag.

Nutrition:

# Baked Red Bell Peppers

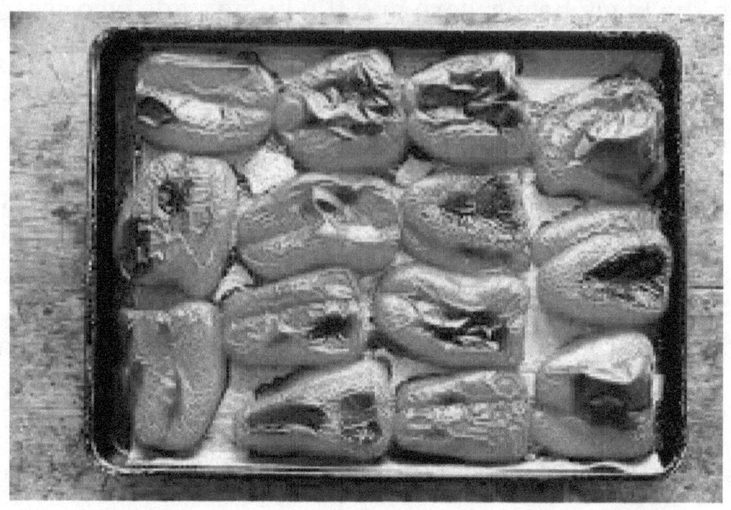

Servings: 8

Preparation Time: 30 minutes

Ingredients :

1 cup dry chickpeas

1½ cup dry quinoa

4 red bell peppers (seeded, halved lengthwise)

1½ tbsp. olive oil

1 red onion (medium, diced)

1 clove garlic (medium, minced)

2 tbsp. chili powder

2 tsp. cumin

1 tsp. cayenne pepper

2 tsp. spicy paprika powder

2 cups baby spinach (chopped)

3 tomatoes (ripe, medium, chopped)

¼ cup fresh cilantro (chopped)

Salt and pepper to taste

Directions:

Preheat the oven to 375°F or 190°C.

Prepare the chickpeas according to the Directions.

Prepare the quinoa according to the recipe.

Put the olive oil into a skillet on medium heat.

Sautee the diced red onions until soft.

Add the garlic, chili powder, cumin, cayenne pepper, paprika powder, salt and pepper to the skillet and stir everything for about 2 minutes.

Stir in the remaining Ingredients except the cilantro and add more salt and pepper to taste.

Heat the stuffing for another 5 minutes until the Ingredients are browned.

Turn off the heat, add dd the cilantro and divide the stuffing into the halved red bell peppers.

Put the peppers on a lightly greased baking tray and cover them with aluminum foil.

Place the tray in the oven for about 20 to 25 minutes.

Take the tray out and allow the bell peppers to sit for about 5 minutes.

Serve right away or allow the stuffed red bell peppers to cool down for storage!

# Quick Quinoa Casserole

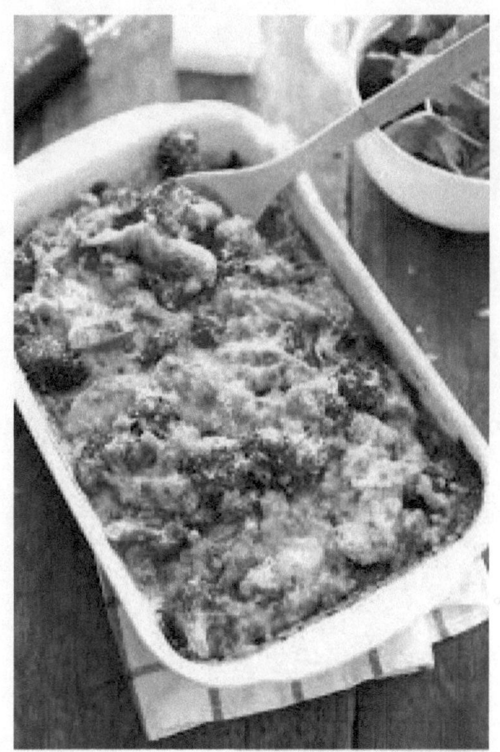

Servings: 9

Preparation Time: 15 minutes

Ingredients :

2 cups dry pinto beans

1 cup dry quinoa

1 (7 oz.) pack tempeh (sliced)

2 tbsp. olive oil

2 tsp. cumin

2 tsp. paprika powder

1 cup red onion (diced)

2 garlic cloves (minced)

6 sweet red peppers (small, sliced)

2 (4 oz.) cans green chilies (diced)

1 cup Roma tomatoes (diced)

2 cups vegetable broth

Salt and pepper to taste

½ cup no-salt cream cheese

1 avocado (diced, sliced or mashed)

¼ cup green onions (diced)

¼ cup cilantro (chopped, fresh)

Directions:

Cook the pinto beans according to the recipe.

Put a large skillet greased with the olive oil over medium heat.

Grill the tempeh slices with a tsp. paprika powder, cumin and salt and pepper to taste for about 5 minutes.

Take out the grilled tempeh slices and leave it aside.

Grease the same skillet with olive oil and sauté the onions.

Add the minced garlic while stirring.

Blend in the red peppers and stir the Ingredients for about 2 minutes.

Continue to add the green chilies, cooked pinto beans and quinoa, tomatoes and vegetable broth to the pan along with another tsp. of paprika powder, cumin, salt and pepper to taste.

Let the mixture cook for about 5 minutes.

Add the tempeh back to the skillet, stir, cover and reduce the heat to low.

Cook the mixture for about 15 minutes until the quinoa is soft and most of the broth has been absorbed.

Remove the skillet from the heat and add vegan cream cheese.

Put the lid on the skillet and let the dish sit for a minute until the cheese has melted.

Serve the quick quinoa casserole with fresh avocado slices, green onions and fresh cilantro.

Enjoy or store!

# Mexican Casserole

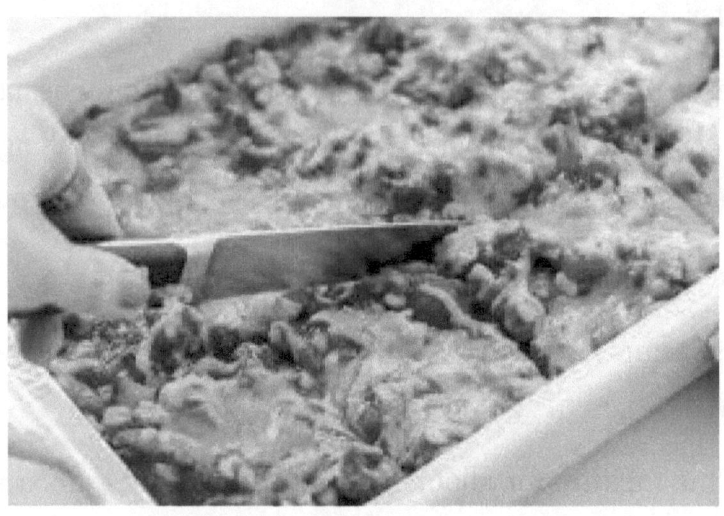

Servings: 4 | Prepping Preparation Time: 30 minutes

Ingredients :

1 cup dry black beans

1 cup dry white beans

1 tsp. olive oil

3 tbsp. Mexican spice

2 cups Mexican salsa

1½ cups cashew cheese spread

3 bell peppers (red and yellow, chopped)

1 red onion (chopped)

1 green onion (chopped)

1 jalapeno pepper (medium, seeded and chopped)

Salt and pepper to taste

Directions:

Cook the beans according to the Directions.

Preheat oven at 350°F or 175°C.

Grease a saucepan with the olive oil. Add Mexican spice, 1 cup of Mexican salsa and stir well.

Stir in the cashew cheese, chopped bell peppers, onions and add salt and pepper to taste.

Spread ½ cup salsa over the bottom of a casserole dish. Add the beans on top of the salsa and spread out the saucepan mix evenly over the beans.

Add the last ½ cup salsa sauce on top and sprinkle some chopped jalapenos on top.

Bake the casserole for 15-20 minutes.

Enjoy the dish after a short cooling period or let it cool down completely for storing.

# Vegan Mac and Cheese

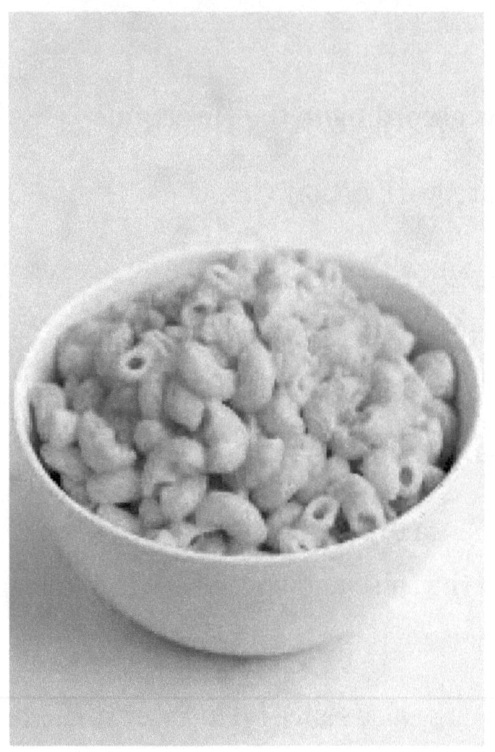

Ingredients :

Cashews (two-thirds cup raw)

Chili flakes (quarter teaspoon)

Nutritional yeast (quarter cup)

Salt and pepper (to taste)

Dry mustard powder (half teaspoon)

Onion powder (half teaspoon)

Garlic powder (half teaspoon)

Garlic (three cloves)

Russet potato (one small)

White onion (one small)

Avocado oil (one and a half tablespoons)

Broccoli (one head)

Apple cider vinegar (two teaspoons)

Macaroni (two cups)

Directions:

Peel and grate potato and grate. Finely dice the garlic.

Heat a large saucepan and oil over medium heat. Put onion and a little salt in the pot and cook until soft.

Put the potato, chili flakes and garlic along with mustard, onion and garlic powders into the pot. Stir well until their flavors release, then add one cup of water and the cashews. Keep stirring at a simmer until the potatoes are soft.

Pour entire mixture into a blender along with the apple cider vinegar and nutritional yeast, then salt and pepper. The consistency should be that of cheese sauce that is thick yet runny. If it is too thick, add more water, if it needs more salt or garlic powder, chili flakes or vinegar, do so now according to your taste.

Put the pasta on the stove in a large pot with water to cover and a little salt. In another pot, boil the broccoli in bite-sized florets until tender.

When both are ready, transfer everything into one pot and cover with the cheese sauce. Combine well, serve and enjoy!

# Mushroom Ragout

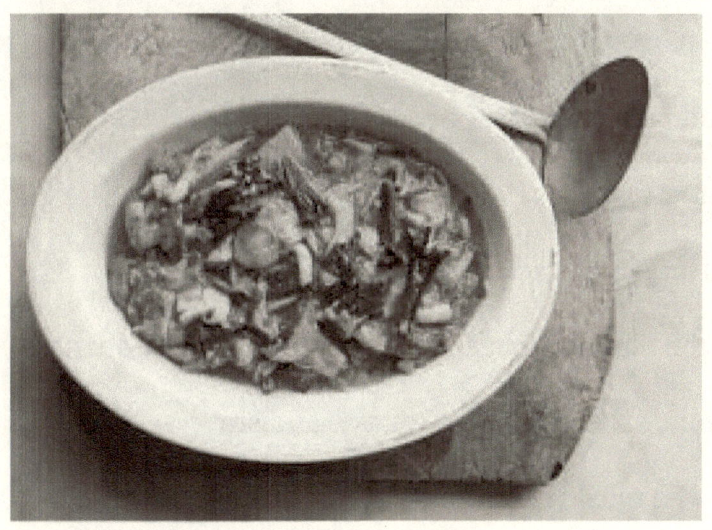

Servings: 10

Preparation Time: 45 min |

Ingredients :

2 tbsp. olive oil

1 sweet onion (large, finely chopped)

1 clove garlic (minced)

6 cups Portobello mushrooms (chopped)

½ cup dry red wine

1 cup vegetable broth

½ tbsp. nutritional yeast

¼ cup basil leaves (chopped)

¼ cup no-salt cream cheese substitute with cashew butter

¼ cup parsley (optional, chopped)

Salt and pepper to taste

Directions:

Take a large pot and put it on medium heat.

Sauté the onions and garlic in the olive oil while stirring.

Add some salt and pepper to taste and stir.

Mix in the mushrooms and turn up the heat a bit.

Cook and stir the mushrooms until most of the liquid in it has evaporated.

Add the red wine. Turn the heat up to medium-high and cook the ragout until most of the wine is evaporated.

Add the vegetable broth and stir thoroughly.

Blend in the nutritional yeast and cook the ragout for about 5 minutes.

Add the chopped basil and the no-salt cream cheese.

Lower the heat and keep stirring until the ragout simmers.

Keep stirring occasionally for about 5 more minutes and add more salt and pepper to taste.

Turn the heat off and set aside for about minutes to let the ragout cool down a bit.

Garnish with the optional parsley before serving and enjoy while warm or store.

# Pumpkin Pilaf

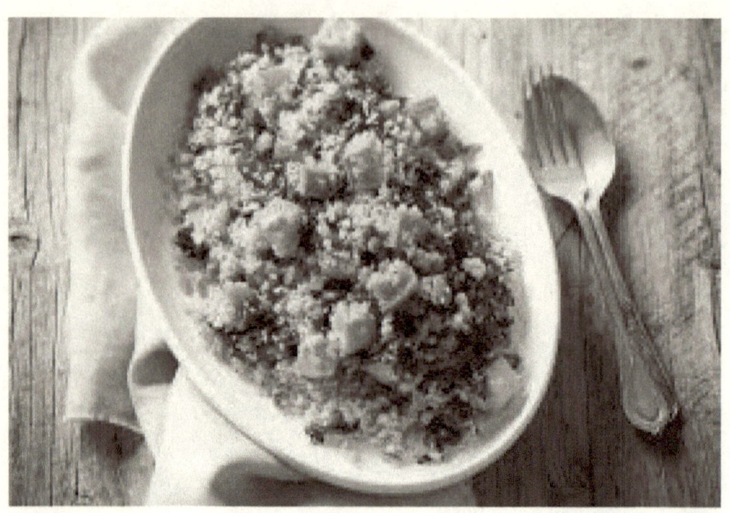

Servings: 2

Preparation Time: 20 minutes

Ingredients :

2 cup dry brown rice

2 tbsp. olive oil

1 sweet potato (medium, cubed)

2 cups fresh pumpkin (cubed)

2 cups kale (fresh or frozen)

2 celery ribs (medium, cut)

1 onion (medium, cut)

2 garlic cloves

1 tbsp. onion powder

1 bay leaf (chopped)

Salt and black pepper to taste

½ cup pumpkin seeds (optional)

Handful of fresh parsley (chopped, optional)

Directions:

Cook the rice according to the recipe.

Put a large skillet on medium heat and add the olive oil to the skillet.

Throw in the sweet potato and pumpkin cubes.

Add the kale, onion, celery, garlic and onion powder.

Cook the mixture for 15-20 minutes and turn the heat down to low.

Add the cooked rice, optional pumpkin seeds, a handful of fresh parsley and stir thoroughly.

Softly cook the mixture for another 5 minutes.

Enjoy or store the pilaf for another day!

# Chapter 9: Desserts and Snacks Recipes

## Sweet Potato Fries

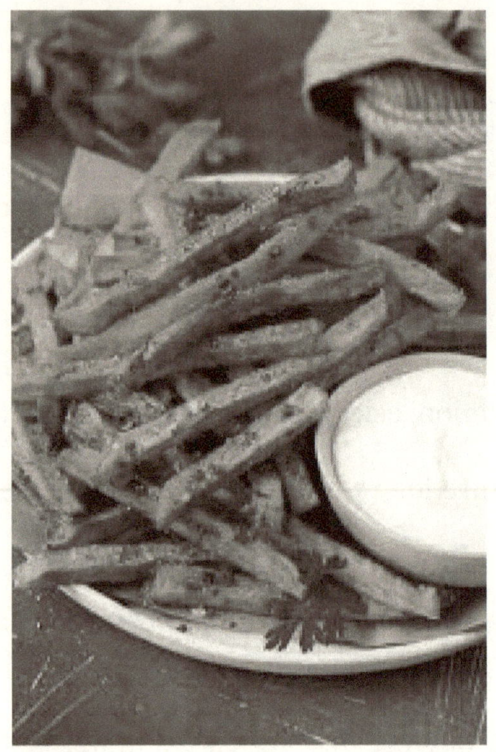

Servings: 2

Preparation Time: 10 minutes

Cooking Time: 25 minutes

Ingredients:

1 large sweet potato, peeled and cut

2 tablespoons extra-virgin oil.

1 teaspoon ground cinnamon

1 teaspoon ground turmeric

Salt and black pepper, to taste

Directions:

Preheat the oven to 425 degrees F and line a baking sheet with foil.

Put all the ingredients in a bowl and toss to coat well.

Spread the mixture on the baking sheet and transfer into the oven.

Bake for 25 minutes and remove from the oven.

Dish out in a platter and serve hot.

# Seed Crackers

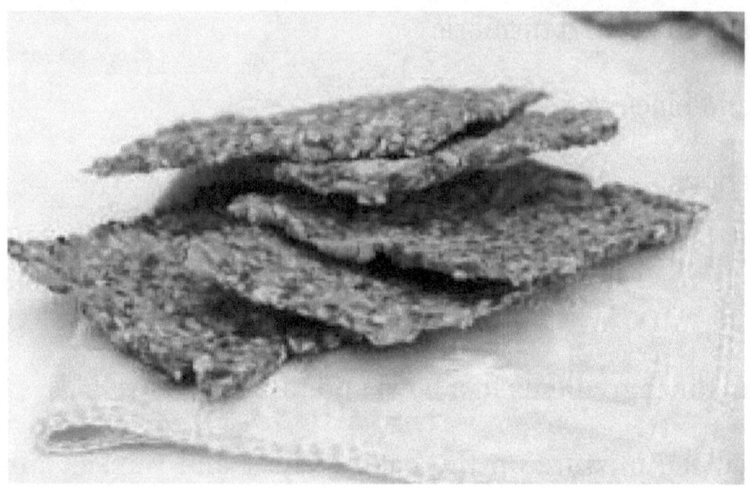

Servings: 6

Preparation Time: 15minutes

Cooking Time: 20 minutes

Ingredients:

3 tablespoons sunflower seeds

1 tablespoon chia seeds

1 teaspoon ground turmeric

3 tablespoons w ater

1 tablespoon quinoa flour

Pinch of salt

Pinch of ground cinnamon

Directions:

Preheat the oven to 345 degrees F and line a baking sheet with the parchment paper.

Add chia seeds in water and soak for 15 minutes.

Add rest of the ingredients and mix well.

Transfer the mixture in the baking tray and spread well.

Cut the shapes of your choice and then transfer into the oven.

Bake for about 20 minutes and remove from the oven.

Allow it to cool down and serve.

# Beet Chips

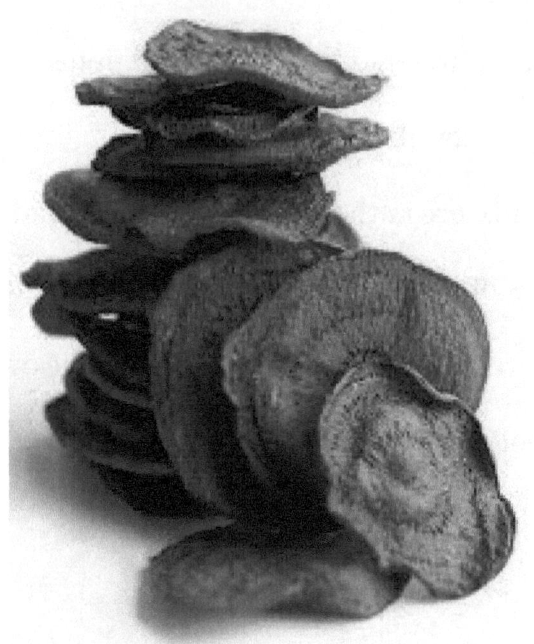

Servings: 6

Preparation  Preparation Time: 10 minutes

Cooking Time: 30 minutes

Ingredients:

1 tablespoon canola oil

2 medium beets, trimmed, peeled, and sliced

Salt, to taste

Directions:

Preheat the oven to 350 degrees F and line 2 large baking sheets along with parchment paper.

Add the beet slices and oil to a bowl and toss well.

Put the beet slices in the baking tray and transfer into the oven.

Bake for 30 minutes and remove from the oven.

Allow it to cool down and serve.

# Cauliflower Popcorn

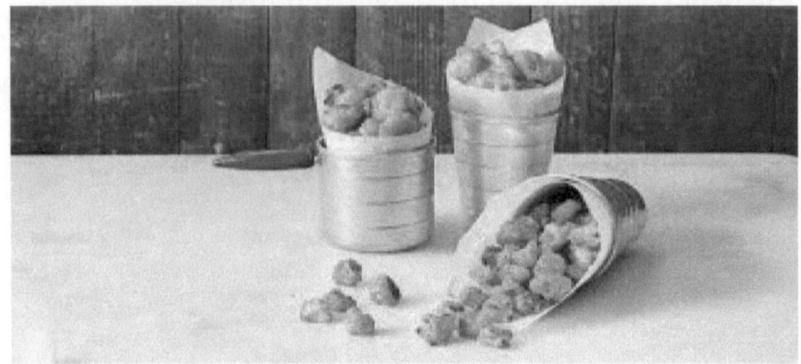

Servings: 6

Preparation Time: 20 minutes

Cooking Time: 30 minutes

Ingredients:

2 teaspoons olive oil

4 cups large cauliflower floret

Salt, as required

Directions:

Preheat the oven to 450 degrees F and grease a roasting pan lightly.

Add all the ingredients to a bowl and toss well.

Transfer this mixture into greased pan and place in the oven.

Roast for about 30 minutes and remove from the oven.

Dish out in a platter and serve immediately.

# Sweetened Pears

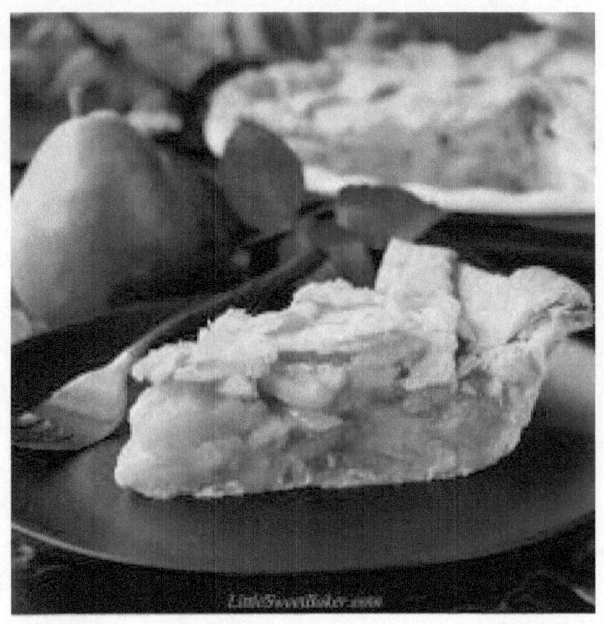

Preparation Time: 10 minutes

Cooking Time: 50 minutes

Servings: 4

Ingredients:

4 pears, peeled

¼ cup sugar

12 oz. dry white wine

1 cinnamon stick

2 tsp. orange zest

1 ½ cups water

½ cup yogurt

1 pod vanilla bean, split

Method:

Use a melon baller to scoop balls from the melons.

Transfer to a bowl and set aside.

In a pan over medium high heat, mix the sugar, wine, cinnamon stick, orange zest and water.

Bring to a boil and simmer until the sugar has dissolved.

Toss the pears in the wine mixture.

Cook for 30 minutes.

Transfer the pears in a bowl.

Cook the syrup for 10 minutes.

Pour the syrup over the pears and serve with yogurt mixed with vanilla.

# Roasted Plums

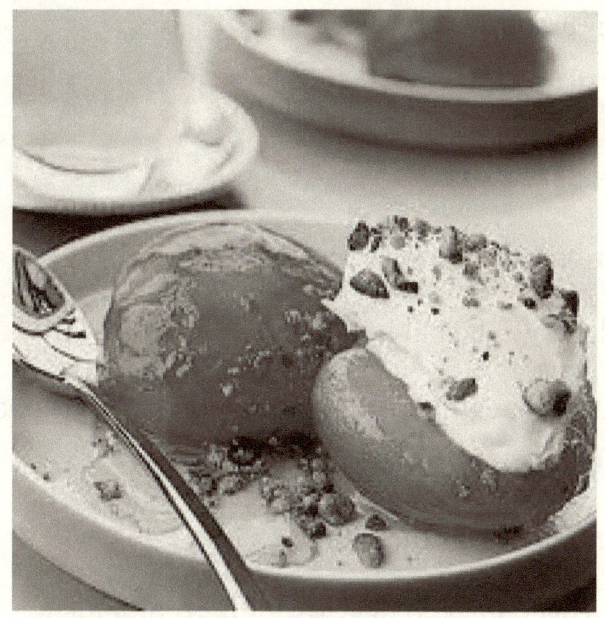

Preparation Time: 10 minutes

Cooking Time: 20 minutes

Servings: 6

Ingredients:

Cooking spray

6 plums, pitted and sliced in half

½ cup pineapple juice

½ tsp. ground cinnamon

3 tbsp. brown sugar, divided

⅛ tsp. ground cumin

¼ tsp. ground cardamom

¼ cup sour cream

2 tbsp. almonds, toasted and slivered

Method:

Spray your baking pan with oil.

Add the plums in the baking pan.

Mix with the pineapple juice, cinnamon, 2 tablespoons sugar, cumin and cardamom.

Pour the mixture over the plums.

Bake in the oven for 450 degrees F for 20 minutes.

In a bowl, mix the sour cream and remaining sugar.

Arrange the roasted plums in a serving bowl.

Top with the sweetened sour cream and almonds.

# Sweetened Mango & Coconut Flakes

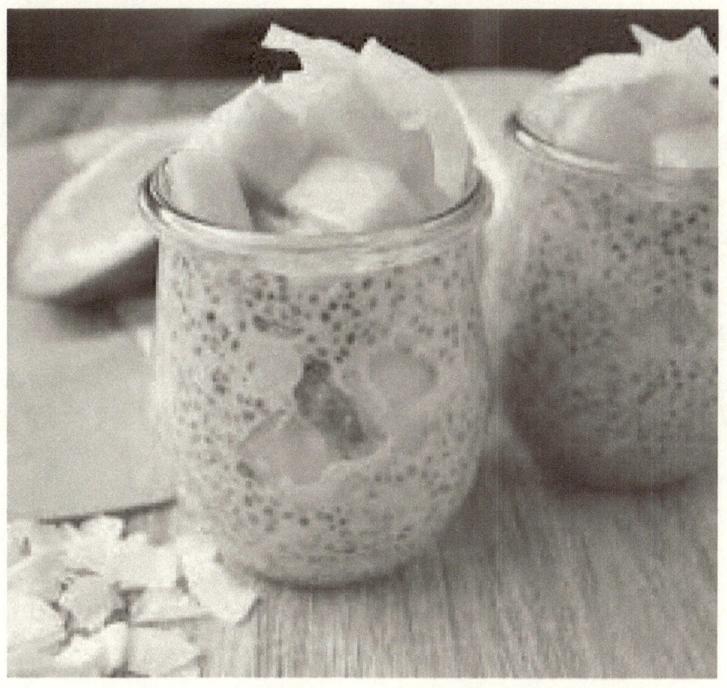

Preparation Time: 10 minutes

Cooking Time: 10 minutes

Servings: 4

Ingredients:

2 mangoes, sliced into cubes

2 tsp. crystallized ginger, chopped

2 tsp. orange zest

2 tbsp. coconut flakes

Method:

Preheat your oven to 350 degrees F.

Add the mangoes to muffin pan.

In a bowl, mix the remaining ingredients and pour over the mangoes.

Roast in the oven for 10 minutes.

# Green Pizza with Bacon

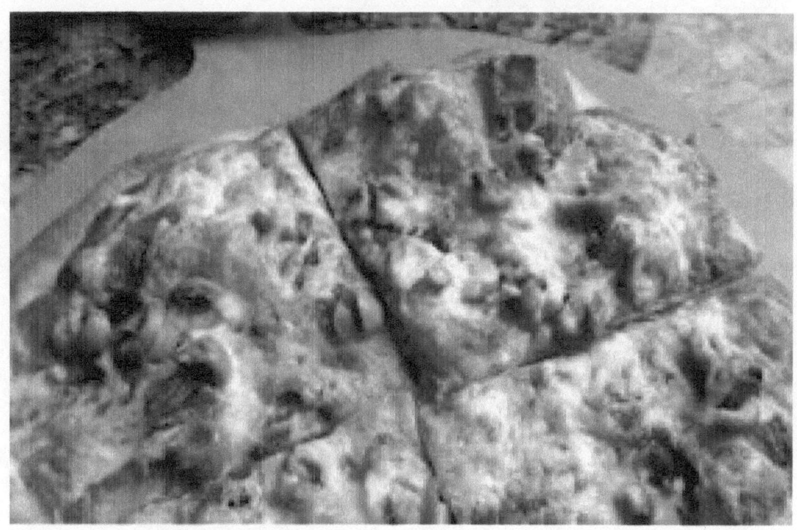

Preparation Time: 10 minutes

Cooking Time: 16 minutes

Servings: 4

Ingredients:

1 whole-wheat pizza crust

½ cup pizza sauce

2 oz. mozzarella cheese

½ cup kale, chopped

4 slices bacon, cooked and sliced

¼ cup pineapple slices

Method:

Preheat your oven to 450 degrees F.

Put the pizza crust on a baking pan and bake for 7 to 8 minutes.

Take it out of the oven and spread pizza sauce on top.

Sprinkle with the cheese, kale, bacon and pineapple slices.

Bake in the oven for another 8 minutes.

# Roasted Vegetables & Sausage Sandwich

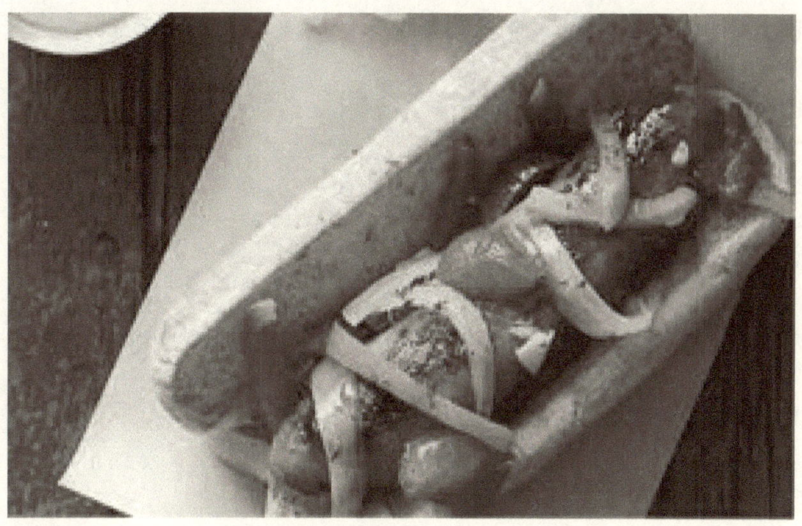

Preparation Time: 15 minutes

Cooking Time: 3 hours and 10 minutes

Servings: 4

Ingredients:

2 tsp. olive oil, divided

2 turkey or chicken sausage links

1 onion, sliced

4 cloves garlic, crushed and minced

1 red bell pepper, sliced

1 cup cherry tomatoes

1 tsp. dried oregano, crushed

2 tsp. honey mustard

3 tbsp. mayonnaise

4 hot dog buns, toasted

Method:

Spray your slow cooker with oil.

Pour half of the olive oil into a pan over medium heat.

Cook the sausage until brown.

Transfer to the slow cooker.

Pour the remaining oil, onion, garlic, bell pepper and tomatoes into the slow cooker.

Season with oregano.

Cover the pot.

Cook on high for 3 hours.

Combine the mustard and mayo in a bowl.

Spread this mixture on the hotdog buns.

Stuff each with the sausage and vegetables.

# Avocado Salad in a Sandwich

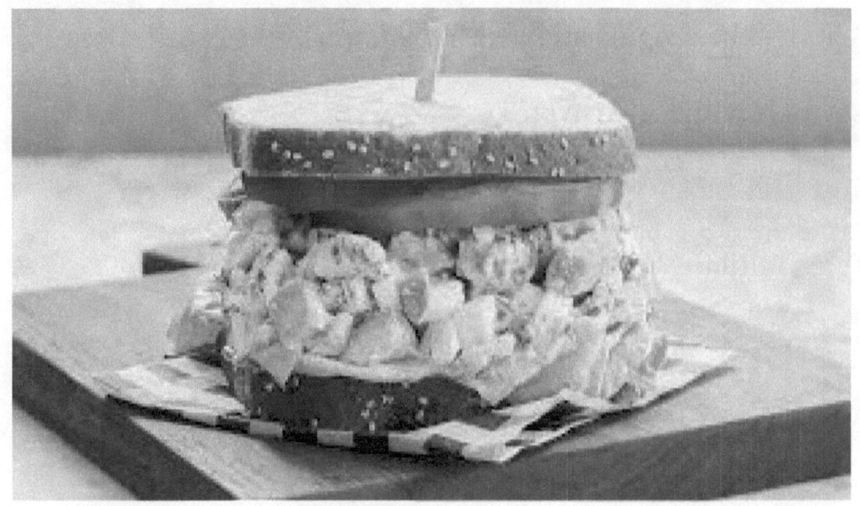

Preparation Time: 10 minutes

Cooking Time: 0 minute

 Servings: 2

Ingredients:

4 whole-wheat bread slices

¼ cup hummus

Pepper to taste

1 cup arugula leaves

½ avocado, sliced

½ cup Gruyere cheese, grated

Method:

Spread each bread slice with hummus and sprinkle with pepper.

Arrange the arugula and avocado on top of the bread slices.

Sprinkle with the Gruyere.

Top with another slice.

Toast until the cheese has melted.

# Vegetable Wraps

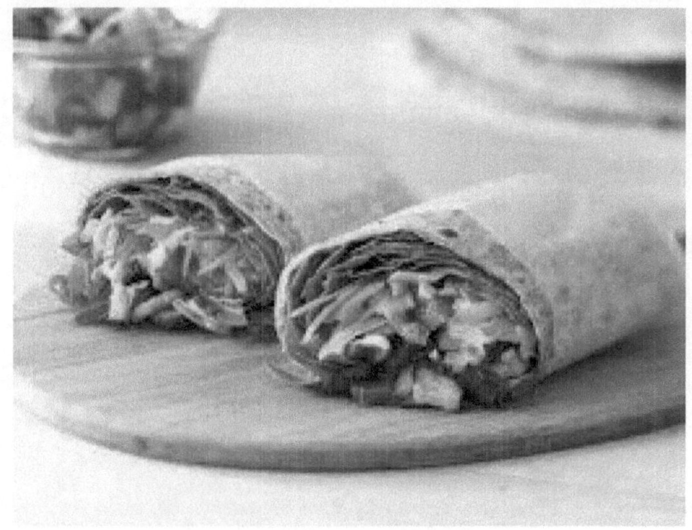

Preparation Time: 10 minutes

Cooking Time: 0 minute

 Servings: 4

Ingredients:

4 tortilla wraps

1 cup hummus

1 cup baby spinach

2 oz. cheddar cheese slices

1 cup red bell pepper, sliced

1 cup broccoli florets, chopped

1 cup carrots, julienned

1 cup red cabbage, shredded

Method:

Spread the tortilla with hummus.

Top with the spinach, cheddar, red bell pepper, broccoli, carrots and cabbage, and roll.

# Turkey Sandwich

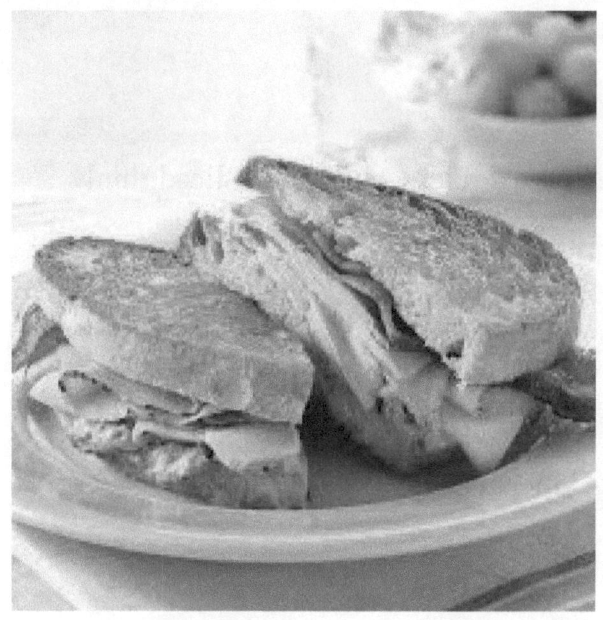

Preparation Time: 15 minutes

Cooking Time: 15 minutes

Servings: 2

Ingredients:

1 tsp. Dijon mustard

1 tbsp. mayonnaise

½ tsp. maple syrup

1 tsp. parsley, chopped

1 tsp. dill, chopped

2 whole-wheat bread slices, toasted

1 tbsp. cold turkey gravy

½ cup lettuce, shredded

¼ avocado, sliced

3 oz. turkey breast fillet, cooked and sliced thinly

1 slice Gouda cheese

2 strips bacon, sliced

1 tsp. olive oil

1 tsp. white vinegar

Pepper to taste

1 tbsp. cranberry sauce

Method:

Mix the mustard, mayo, maple syrup, parsley and dill in a bowl.

Spread one bread slice with this mixture.

Top it with gravy.

Arrange the lettuce, avocado, turkey and cheese on top.

Drizzle with the oil, vinegar and season with pepper.

Spread the cranberry sauce on top of the other bread slice and place this on top of the sandwich.

# Garlic Mashed Potatoes

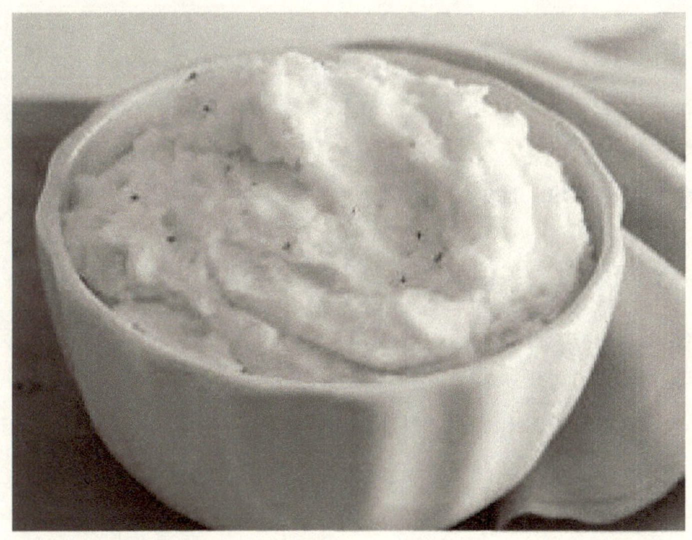

Preparation Time: 20 minutes

Cooking Time: 10 minutes

Servings: 4

Ingredients:

2 lb. potatoes, sliced into cubes

6 cloves garlic

Salt and pepper to taste

½ cup chicken broth

2 tbsp. sour cream

Pinch nutmeg

Method:

Add the garlic and potatoes in a pot with water.

Season with salt.

Cover the pot.

Boil until potatoes are tender.

Drain the potatoes and mash with fork or potato masher.

Stir in broth and add the sour cream.

Season with nutmeg, salt and pepper.

# Green Beans with Roasted Red Peppers

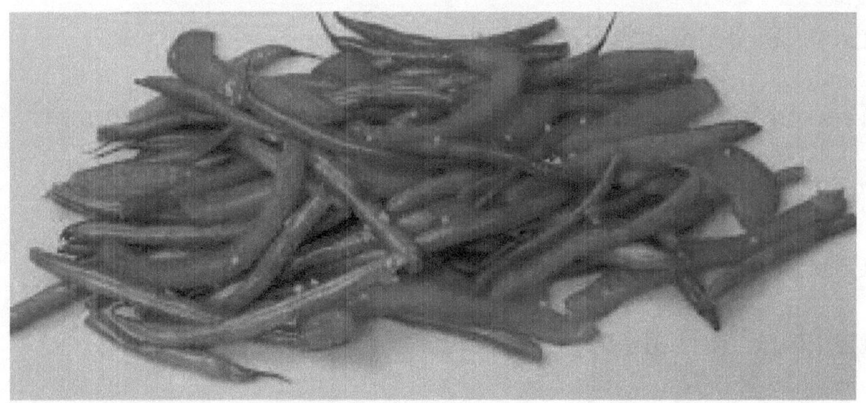

Preparation Time: 10 minutes

Cooking Time: 12 minutes

Servings: 6

Ingredients:

1 tbsp. olive oil

1 cup onion, chopped

1 tbsp. balsamic vinegar

½ cup roasted red pe ppers, chopped

¼ cup olives, pitted and sliced

2 tbsp. fresh basil, chopped

Salt and pepper to taste

1 lb. green beans, sliced and steamed

Method:

Pour the oil into a pan over medium heat.

Cook the onion for 10 minutes.

Pour in the vinegar and cook for 2 minutes, stirring frequently.

Add the olives, red peppers, salt, pepper and basil.

Cook for 2 minutes and remove from heat.

Combine the red pepper mixture and green beans.

# Zucchini Fries & Dip

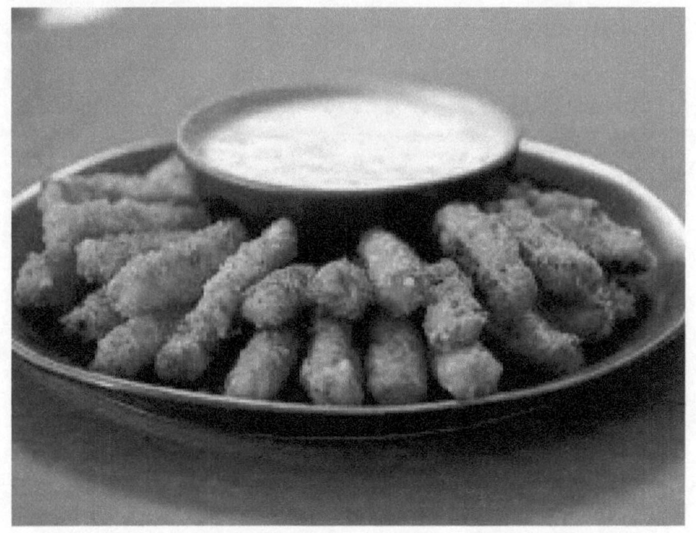

Preparation Time: 20 minutes

Cooking Time: 30 minutes

Servings: 6

Ingredients:

Cooking spray

1 zucchini, sliced into strips

2 eggs

1 tbsp. water

¾ whole-wheat breadcrumbs

2 tsp. Old Bay seasoning

Pepper to taste

1 tbsp. lemon juice

2 tbsp. mayonnaise

¼ cup Greek yogurt

½ tsp. garlic powder

 Salt to taste

1/8 cup chives, chopped

1/8 cup parsley, chopped

Method:

Preheat your oven to 425 degrees F.

Spray a baking pan with oil.

Mix the eggs and water in a bowl.

Add the breadcrumbs, Old Bay seasoning and pepper in another bowl.

Dip the zucchini strips in the first and second bowls.

Arrange on the baking pan.

Bake for 30 minutes.

Mix the rest of the ingredients in a dipping bowl.

Serve the fries with the dip.

# Roasted Mushrooms

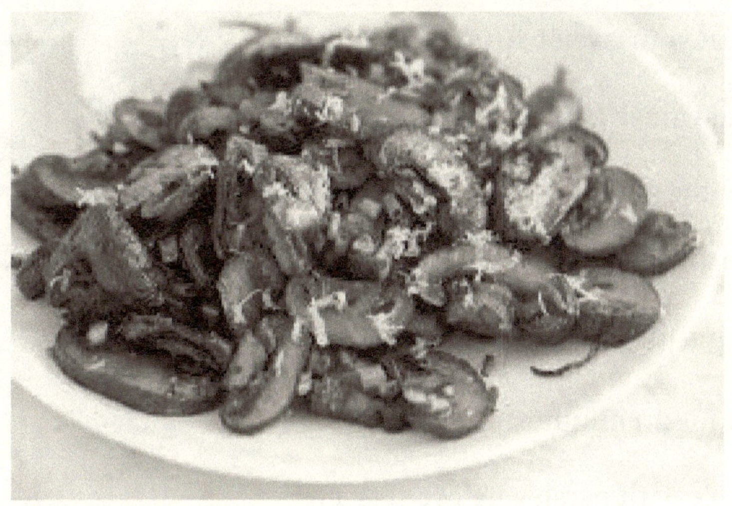

Preparation Time: 15 minutes

Cooking Time: 20 minutes

Servings: 6

Ingredients:

1 lb. fresh mushrooms, sliced

6 cloves garlic, sliced

2 tbsp. olive oil

2 tsp. balsamic vinegar

2 tsp. Worcestershire sauce

1 tsp. dried oregano

Salt and pepper to taste

2 tbsp. parsley, chopped

Method:

Preheat your oven to 400°F.

Add the mushrooms on a baking pan.

Stir in the garlic.

Drizzle the top with oil, vinegar, and Worcestershire sauce.

Season with salt, pepper and oregano.

Roast for 20 minutes.

Sprinkle with parsley before serving.

# Roasted Brussels Sprouts

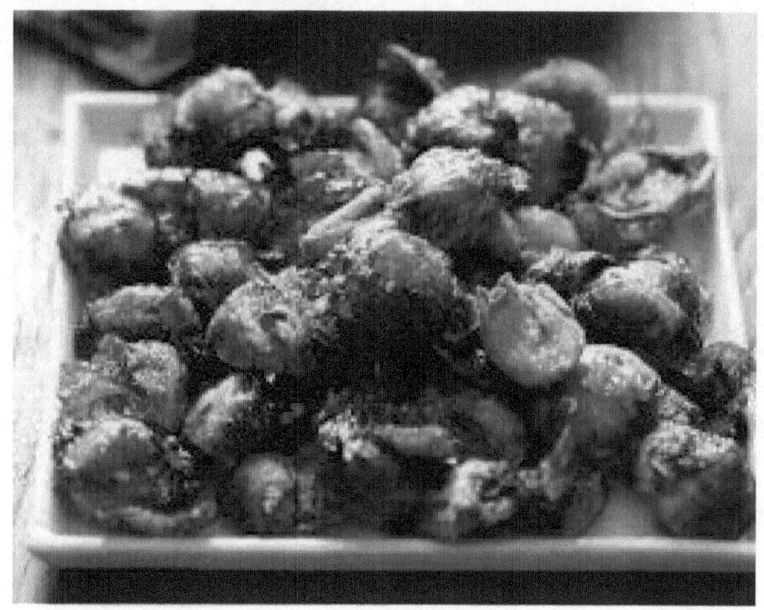

Preparation Time: 10 minutes

Cooking Time: 15 minutes

Servings: 4

Ingredients:

Cooking spray

1 lb. Brussels sprouts, sliced in half

1 tsp. olive oil

Salt and pepper to taste

1 tbsp. lemon juice

Method:

Preheat your oven to 425 degrees F.

Line your baking sheet with foil.

Spray with oil.

Toss the Brussels sprouts in oil and season with salt and pepper.

Roast for 15 minutes.

Drizzle with lemon juice before serving.

# Fruit Compote

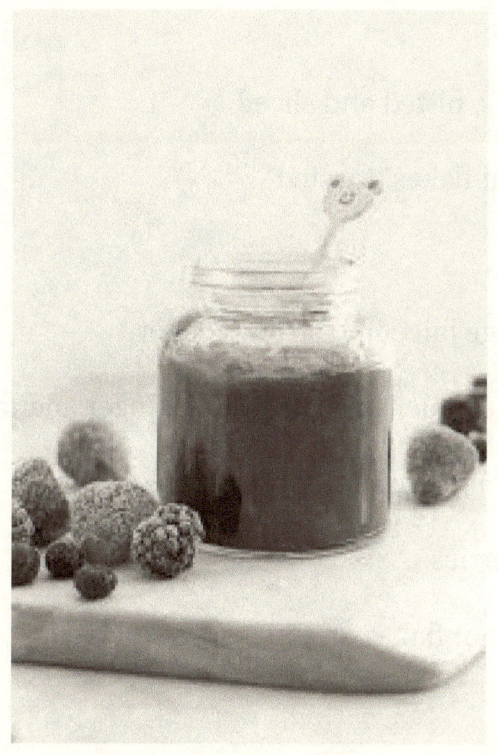

Preparation Time: 10 minutes

Cooking Time: 8 minutes

Servings: 10

Ingredients:

3 tbsp. orange juice

15 oz. pineapple chunks

¾ cup dried apricots, sliced into quarters

3 pears, sliced into cubes

1 tsp. ginger, grated

1 tbsp. tapioca

2 cups cherries, pitted and sliced

¼ cup coconut flakes, toasted

Method:

Pour the orange juice into a slow cooker.

Stir in the pineapple, apricots, pears, ginger and tapioca.

Cover the pot and cook for 8 hours on low setting.

Stir in the cherries.

Sprinkle coconut flakes on top before serving.

# Figs with Walnuts, Honey & Yogurt

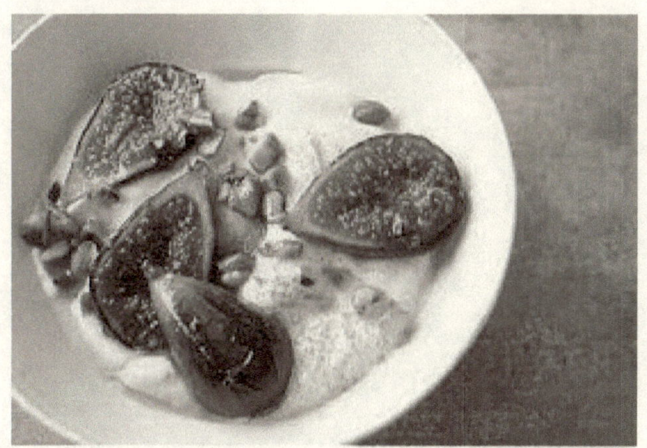

Preparation Time: 5 minutes

Cooking Time: 0 minute

 Servings: 4

Ingredients:

2 figs, sliced

2 tsp. honey

½ tsp. vanilla

8 oz. yogurt, refrigerated for 8 hours

1 tbsp. walnuts, chopped and toasted

Method:

Combine all the ingredients except walnuts in a serving bowl.

Sprinkle the walnuts on top.

# Yogurt Strawberries

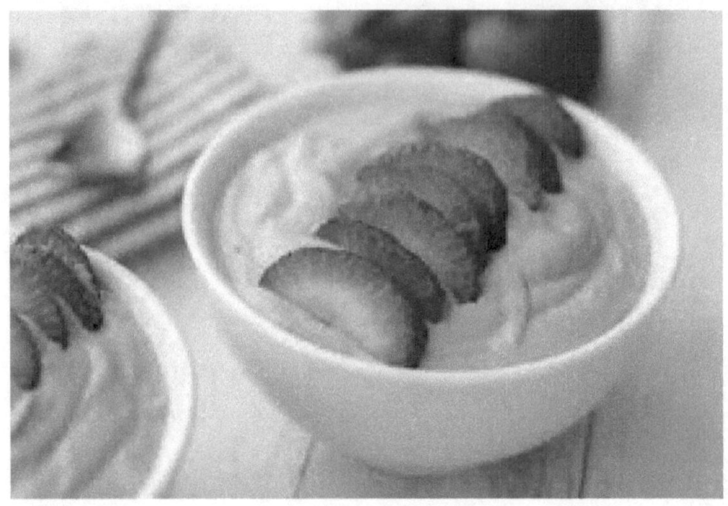

Preparation Time: 1 hour and 5 minutes

Cooking Time: 0 minute

 Servings: 1

Ingredients:

3 strawberries, sliced

1 tbsp. plain Greek yogurt

Method:

Combine the strawberries and yogurt.

Refrigerate for 1 hour.

Nutritional Value:

# Celery Crackers

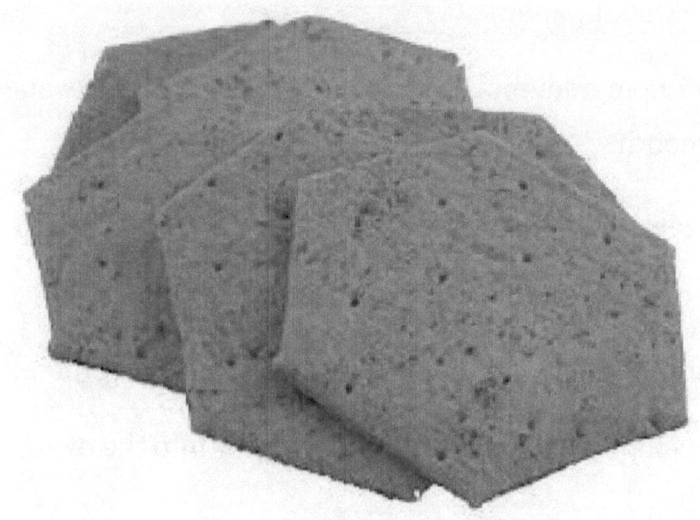

Servings: 15

Preparation Time: 10 minutes

Cooking Time: 2 hours Ingredients:

3 cups flax seeds, ground

10 celery sticks

¼ cup coconut oil

1 teaspoon fresh thyme leaves

1 teaspoon fresh rosemary  leaves

2 tablespoons apple cider vinegar

Salt, to taste

Directions:

Preheat the oven to 225 degrees F and line 2 baking sheets with the parchment paper.

Add all the ingredients to a blender except flax seeds and blend until smooth.

Add the flax seeds and pulse well to form dough.

Take it out in a bowl and divide into two halves.

Place both halves onto the baking sheets and press them.

Cut the shapes of your choice and transfer into the oven.

Bake for about 1 hour on each side and remove from the oven.

Allow it to cool down and serve.

# Veggie Bites

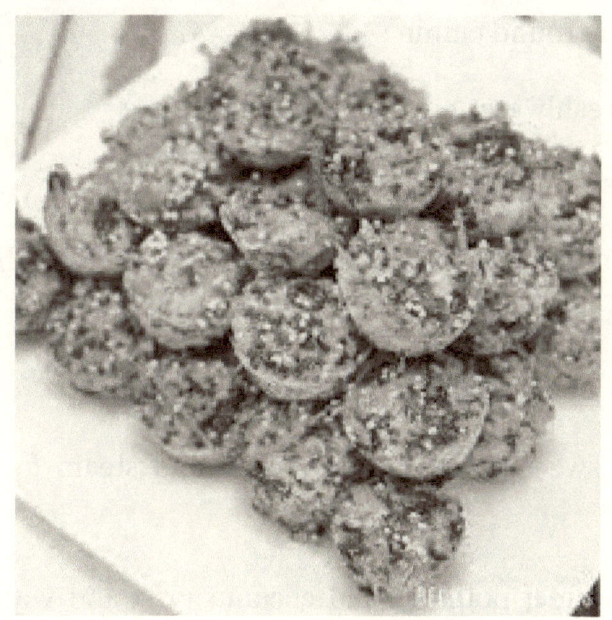

Servings: 6

Preparation Time: 15 minutes

Cooking Time: 25 minutes

Ingredients:

1 medium shallot, chopped

2 medium sweet potatoes, peeled and cubed

2 tablespoons coconut milk

1 cup fresh kale leaves, toug h ends removed and chopped

½ teaspoon granulated garlic

¼ teaspoon ground turmeric

ground flaxseeds, as needed

1 teaspoon ground cumin

Salt and freshly ground black pepper, to taste

Directions:

Preheat the oven to 400 degrees F and line a baking sheet with a parchment paper.

Arrange a steamer basket in a pan of water.

Place the sweet potato in the basket and steam for about 15 minutes.

Mash the sweet potatoes and coconut milk and with a potato masher.

Add rest of the ingredients to the potatoes except flaxseeds.

Prepare small balls from the mixture and arrange on the baking tray.

Sprinkle with flaxseeds and bake for about 25 minutes.

Remove from the oven and serve immediately.

# Peanut Butter Bites

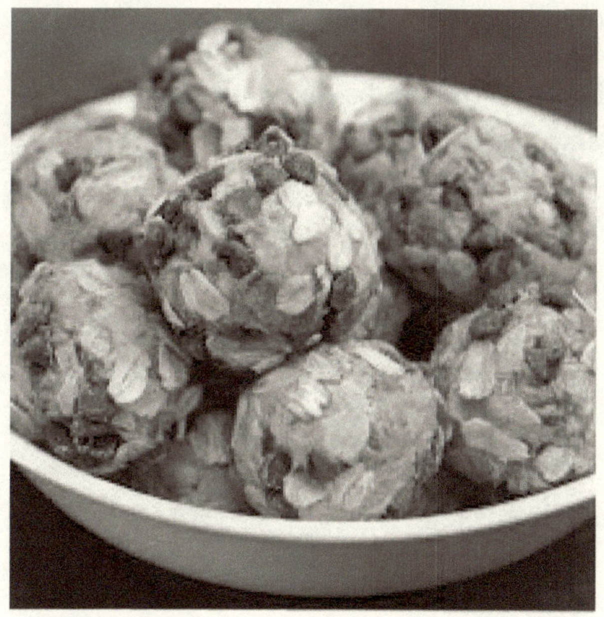

Servings: 10

Preparation Time: 40 minutes

Ingredients:

½ cup coconut flour

1/3 cup maple syrup

1 cup creamy peanut butter, unsalted

Directions:

Put all the ingredients in a bowl and whisk to form a thick mixture.

Wrap the bowl and freeze for about 20 minutes.

Remove from the freezer and make small balls from the mixture using a cookie scooper.

Arrange the balls on the baking tray and freeze for about 20 minutes before serving.

# Grilled Peaches

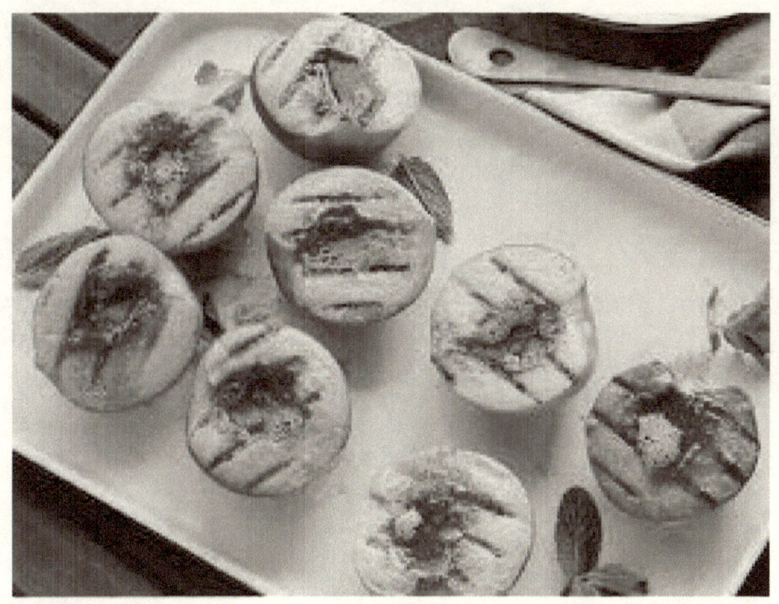

Servings: 4

Preparation  Preparation Time: 10 minutes

Cooking Time: 5 minutes

Ingredients:

2 large peaches, halved and pitted

¼ teaspoon cinnamon, ground

1 teaspoon vanilla extract

¼ cup coconut cream

1 teaspoon sugar, powdered

Directions:

Preheat the grill to medium-high heat and grease the grill grate.

Place the peach halves onto the prepared grill by adjusting the cut side down and grill for about 5 minutes.

Add the coconut cream, sugar and vanilla extract in a bowl and beat well.

Remove the peach halves from the grill and serve topped with coconut cream and cinnamon.

# Oat Stuffed Pears

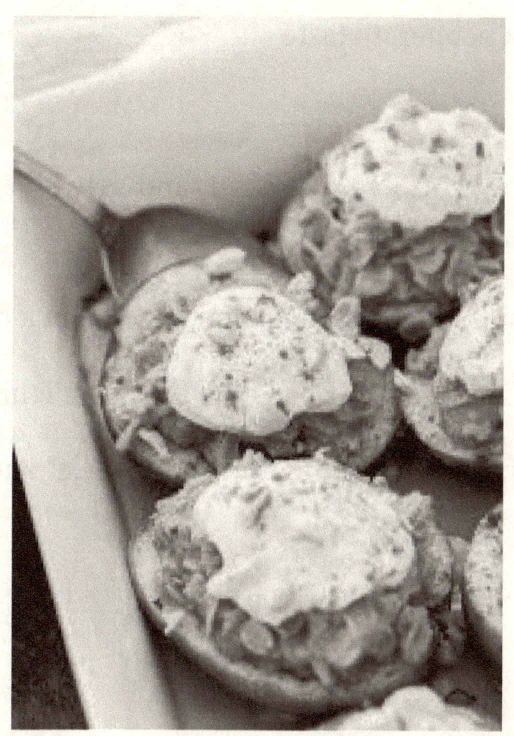

Servings: 4

Preparation Time: 10minutes

Cooking Time: 25 minutes

Ingredients:

4 tablespoons Parmesan cheese, grated

2 cups vegetable broth

6 tablespoons lemon juice

2 teaspoons fresh lemon zest, grated

2 cups white rice, rinsed

4 tablespoons fresh mint leaves, chopped

Salt and black pepper, to taste

Directions:

Preheat the oven to 375 degrees F and grease a baking sheet lightly.

Mix oats, raisins, almonds, cinnamon and oil in a bowl.

Fill the oat mixture in pear halves, and press slightly.

Arrange the pear halves onto the baking sheet and bake for 25 minutes

Drizzle with maple syrup and serve warm.

# Strawberry Ice-cream

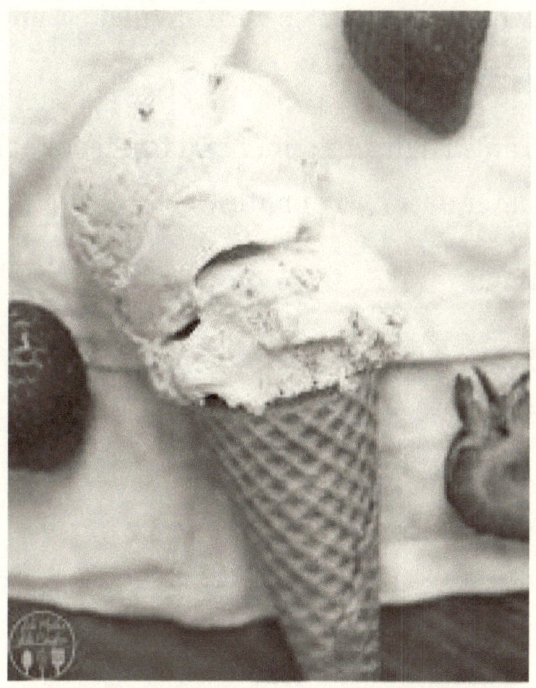

Servings: 4

Preparation Time: 15minutes

Ingredients:

2 tablespoons coconut, shredded

1 cup fresh strawberries, hulled an d sliced

½ small banana, peeled and sliced

½ cup coconut cream

Directions:

Add all the ingredients to a high speed blender and blend until smooth.

Pour the mixture into the ice-cream maker and process as dictated in instructions.

Transfer into an airtight container and freeze for at least 4 hours with stirring after every 30 minutes.

Serve and enjoy!

# Berries Granita

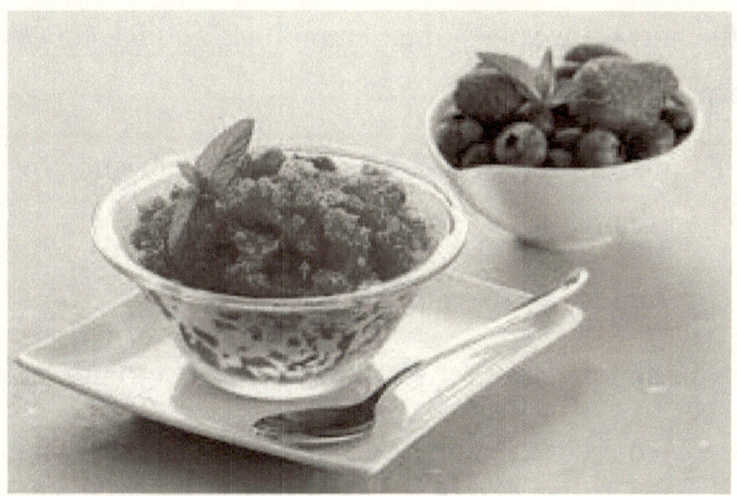

Servings: 4

Preparation Time: 4 hours Ingredients:

½ cup fresh strawberries, hulled and sliced

½ cup fresh blackberries

½ cup fresh blueberries

½ cup fresh raspberries

1 teaspoon fresh mint leaves

1 tablespoon fresh lemon juice

1 tablespoon maple syrup

¼ cup coconut cream

2-3 drops liquid stevia

1 cup ice-cubes, crushed

Directions:

Add the berries, maple syrup, lemon juice and ice cubes into a blender and blend well.

Put this mixture into an 8x8-inch baking dish and freeze for about 30 minutes.

Take out from the freezer and stir well.

Freeze for about 3 hours and scrape after every 30 minutes.

Add the coconut cream and stevia to a bowl and form foam.

Place the granita into serving glasses and serve topped with coconut cream and mint leaves.

## Coffee Jelly

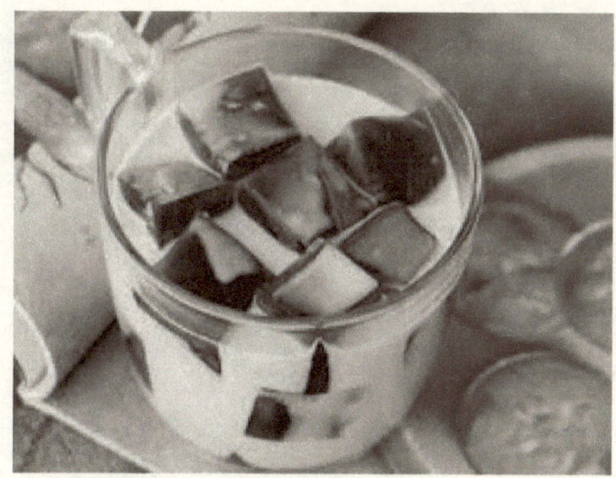

Servings: 4

Preparation Time: 20 minutes

Ingredients:

2 cups coffee, brewed

1 tablespoon vegan gelatin powder

3 tablespoons sugar

4 tablespoons water

Directions:

Dissolve the gelatin powder in water.

Boil coffee and sugar in a pan.

Remove from the heat and stir in the gelatin mixture with constant stirring.

Refrigerate to cool before serving.

# Chocolaty Tofu Mousse

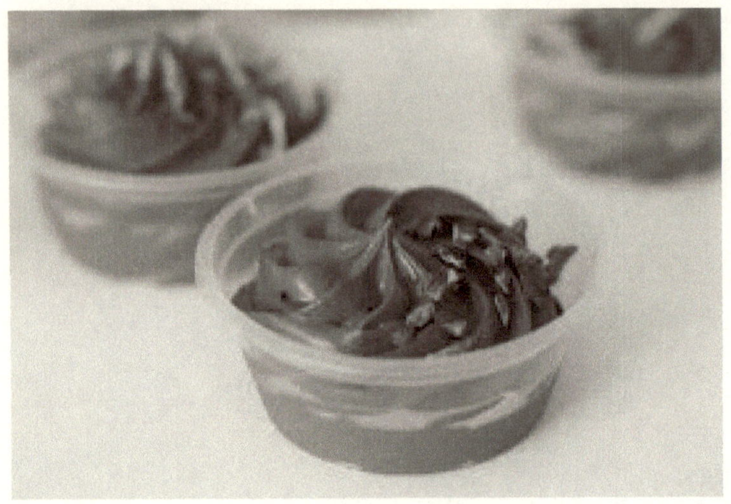

Servings: 4

Preparation Time: 15 minutes

Ingredients:

10 drops liquid stevia

2 cups tofu, drained

1 tablespoon vanilla extract

2 tablespoons cocoa powder

¼ cup almond milk

Directions:

Put all the ingredients in a blender and blend until smooth.

Transfer into serving bowls and chill before serving.

# Gluten Free Crackers

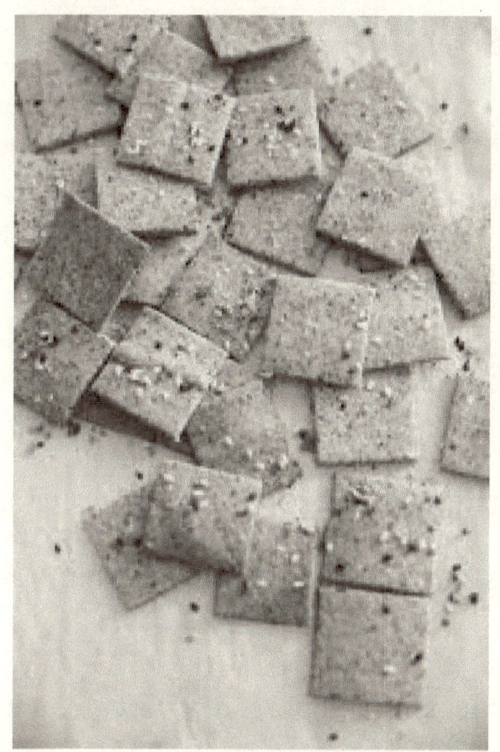

Servings: 4

Preparation Time:10 minutes

Cooking Time: 20 minutes

Ingredients:

¼ teaspoon paprika, sm oked

¼ teaspoon onion, powdered

¼ teaspoon garlic, powdered

1 cup all-purpose flour

½ teaspoon xanthan gum

¼ teaspoon sea salt

¼ cup water

½ teaspoon baking powder

1 teaspoon sugar

¼ cup butter, chilled and diced

Directions:

Whisk all the ingredients in a bowl except water and butter.

Add the cubes butter to the flour blend and form a dough by adding water.

Take it out of the bowl and prepare a disk out of it.

Put it back in the bowl and refrigerate for about 10 minutes.

Preheat the oven to 450 degrees F and grease a baking tray lightly.

Spread the dough between two parchment papers and roll it to obtain a thickness of 1.8 inches.

Remove the parchment paper at the top.

Cut into squares and place them in the baking tray.

Bake for about 20 minutes and dish out to serve.

# Strawberry Short Cakes

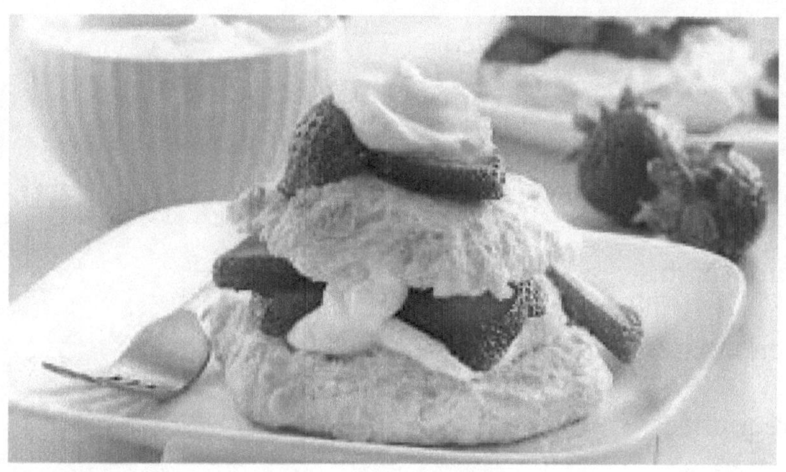

Servings: 9

Preparation Time: 15 minutes

Cooking Time: 20 minutes

Ingredients: For the Shortcake:

2 tablespoons lemon juice

3 cups self-rising flour

½ cup vegan butter

¾ cup soy milk

½ teaspoon salt

1 teaspoon vanilla extract

1 teaspoon baking powder

¼ cup caster sugar

For the Vegan Whipped Cream:

1 can coconut cream, chilled

3 tablespoons vegan sugar

For the Strawberries:

3 cups fresh strawberries, sliced

¼ cup caster sugar

Directions:

Preheat the oven to 450 degrees F.

Sift the salt along baking powder in the flour.

Add vegan butter to the flour bowl and mix with hands.

Add in sugar.

Mix the buttermilk, soy milk, and lemon juice.

Add it to the dry mixture.

Mix vanilla to the ingredients.

Flour a surface and form a smooth dough out of it.

Cut cakes out of the dough by using a cutter.

Line a baking tray with parchment paper and place these cakes onto it.

Brush soy milk on the top of shortcakes.

Bake in the oven for 20 minutes.

Cut the strawberries into slices, dip them in sugar, and refrigerate.

Whip coconut cream using an electric whisk to obtain whipped cream.

Add in the powdered sugar and whip again.

Slice the baked cakes, fill them with cream and strawberry slices.

Enjoy with family!

# 5 Minutes Pancakes

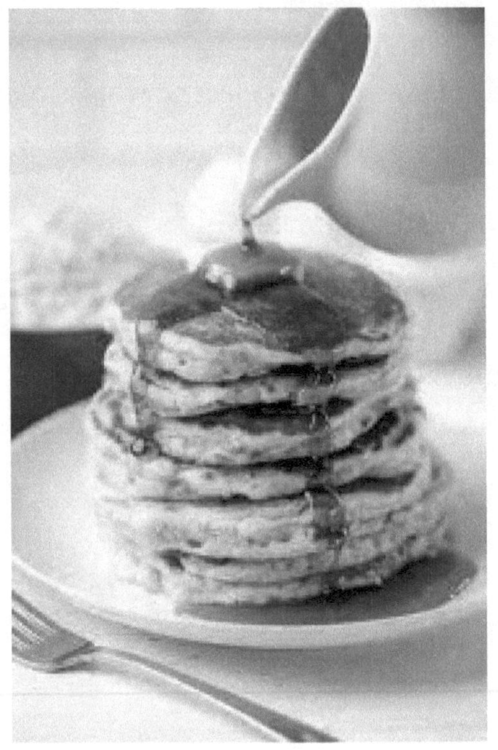

Servings: 2

Preparation Time: 5 minutes

Cooking Time: 15 minutes

Ingredients:

1/8 teaspoon salt

2 tablespoons baking powder

1 cup soymilk

1 cup flour

1 tablespoon sugar

2 tablespoons vegetable oil

Directions:

Turn on the flame and bring it to medium heat.

Take a bowl, add flour, sugar, baking powder, and salt to it and mix them.

Add vegetable oil and soy milk to the bowl with dry mixture and mix well until smooth.

Spoon out the batter in the pan set on heat.

Flip the cakes when they are cooked from one side.

Remove from heat when cooked.

Enjoy with jam or anything that you like.

# Green Pea Guacamole

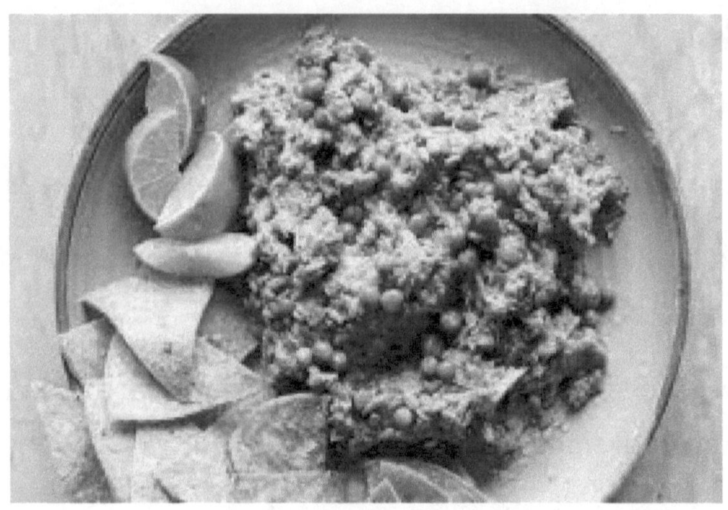

Servings: 4

Preparation Time: 35 minutes

Ingredients:

1 tomato, chopped

1 teaspoon garlic, crushed

½ cup fresh cilantro, chopped

Sea salt, to taste

¼ cup fresh lime juice

4 green onions, chopped

2 cups frozen green peas, thawed

½ teaspoon ground cumin

⅛ teaspoon hot sauce

Directions:

Put the peas, lime juice, garlic, and cumin in a food processor and process until smooth.

Dish out the mixture into a bowl and add green onion, tomato, hot sauce, and cilantro.

Season with salt and cover the bowl.

Refrigerate for about 30 minutes and serve chilled.

# Chapter 10:  4 Weeks Plant Based Meal Plan

| DAYS | BREAKFAST | LUNCH/DINNER | SNACKS/DESSERT |
|---|---|---|---|
| 1 | Tropi-Kale Breeze | Banh Mi | Sweet Potato Fries |
| 2 | Tofu-Spinach Scramble | Sweet Potato Buddha Bowl Almond Butter Dressing | Seed Crackers |
| 3 | Chai Chia Smoothie | Curry Spiced Sweet Potato Wild Rice Burgers | Beet Chips |
| 4 | Banana Bread Rice Pudding | Calabacitas Quesadillas | Cauliflower Popcorn |
| 5 | Broiled Grapefruit with Cinnamon Pitas | Chickpea Avocado Salad Sandwich With Cranberries | Sweetened Pears |

| 6 | Chocolate PB Smoothie | Rice Paper Rolls with Mango and Mint | Sweetened Mango & Coconut Flakes |
|---|---|---|---|
| 7 | Orange French Toast | Turmeric Chickpea Salad Sandwich | Green Pizza with Bacon |
| 8 | Oatmeal Raisin Breakfast Cookie | Mexican Quinoa | Roasted Vegetables & Sausage Sandwich |
| 9 | Berry Beetsicle Smoothie | Potato Fritters | Vegetable Wraps |
| 10 | Blueberry Oat Muffins | Broccoli Pesto with Pasta and Cherry Tomatoes | Turkey Sandwich |
| 11 | Quinoa Applesauce Muffins | Korean Barbecue Tempeh Wraps | Garlic Mashed Potatoes |
| 12 | Pumpkin Pancakes | Crab Cakes | Zucchini Fries & Dip |

| 13 | Green Breakfast Smoothie | Smoky Black Beans Parsley Chimichurri | Roasted Mushrooms |
|---|---|---|---|
| 14 | Blueberry Lemonade Smoothie | Tuna Sandwich With Chickpeas | Roasted Brussels Sprouts |
| 15 | Berry Protein Smoothie | Sweet Potato Toast | Fruit Compote |
| 16 | Flaxseed Porridge | Cucumber Avocado Toast | Figs with Walnuts, Honey & Yogurt |
| 17 | Spicy Hash Browns | Tofu Fish Sticks | Yogurt Strawberries |
| 18 | Kiwi Slushie | Baked Sweet Potato Fries | Celery Crackers |
| 19 | Chia Seed Smoothie | Butternut Squash Linguine With Fried Sage | Veggie Bites |
| 20 | Mango Smoothie | Chickpea Biryani | Peanut Butter Bites |
| 21 | Quinoa & Chocolate Bowl | Chinese Eggplant | Grilled Peaches |

| 22 | Vegetable Hash | Spaghetti Alla Puttanesca | Oat Stuffed Pears |
|---|---|---|---|
| 23 | Walnut Porridge | Thai Red Curry | Strawberry Ice-cream |
| 24 | Granola | Tamarind Potato Curry | Berries Granita |
| 25 | Breakfast Cereal | Kale Slaw | Coffee Jelly |
| 26 | Fruity Oatmeal | Moroccan Veggie Soup | Chocolaty Tofu Mousse |
| 27 | Pecan Pumpkin Spice Oatmeal | Lentil Fattoush Salad | Gluten Free Crackers |
| 28 | Carrot Cake Oatmeal with Cream Cheese Frosting | Sweet Potato Salad | Strawberry Short Cakes |

# Conclusion

Plants are a good source of all nutrients and minerals. They have low cholesterol, good lipids, and antioxidant characteristics which help to detoxify the body from pollutants. A plant-based diet has a significant impact on health, skin, and the environment. Plant-based diet improves and provides shine to the skin. This book is a complete guide for beginners who intend to reduce weight, strengthen muscles and bones, and health-related problems such as heart diseases, obesity, and metabolic syndromes.

Enjoy this book with all vegan recipes and 28-days meal plan, which will help you to decide your daily food.